KILLING FAT

A WEIGHT LOSS JOURNEY AND ACTION PLAN FOR YOUR PATH TO A HEALTHIER LIFE

DEREK A COX

WHY I WROTE THIS BOOK

I wrote this book because I want to share my story with you, create a connection with and become your friend. I am writing out of a love and desire to help people with their weight loss and fitness goals. As your friend I want to show you a path you can take and encourage you along the way. When you fall off the bandwagon like I have, I want to be that friend who helps you back up with encouragement.

I want to share with you that I have been through it myself, felt the same physical & emotinal pains of being obese, and have found the motivation to reach the other side.

To tell you the truth, I have put off writing this book for many years and even tried to get out of writing it all together. You see, I have never seen myself as a writer but I do really enjoy talking to people and encourageing them and God has put it on my heart to help as many people as I can.

There is a quote by Erma Bombeck, "When I stand before God at the end of my life, I would hope that I would not have a single bit of talent left, and could say, 'I used everything you gave me'."

This quote brings tears to eyes everytime I read it and is one of my motivation pieces in bringing this book to you and providing as much help to as many people as I can no matter if it is weight loss, improving mobility or training for a sport.

WHY YOU SHOULD READ THIS BOOK

According to the Center for Disease Control and Prevention (CDC), in 2013 there where over 78 million Adults suffering from obesity and over 12 million children suffering as well.

This book will help you escape those statistics

We will go through some of the emotions and physical pains.

Help you in finding your motivation and defining your goals.

We will start to change your patterns while briefly going over the health benefits of exercise and physical activity

We will touch on nutrition basics and recommendations helping you break out of the bad habit cycles and replacing them with good habits.

This book will also help you build your exercise plan making the most of your time and show you how to track your progress to look back on for more motivation.

There will be action steps along the way and a link provided to **Download a Free PDF** workbook for your convenience in following the action steps.

Acknowledgements

I would like to express my gratitude to the people who contributed to this book as well as those who supported and encouraged and corrected me.

First a Big thank you to my wife Annie without your love or the constant encouragement you have provided me, this book would have only been stories and advice I tell my friends randomly instead of a dream completed.

To my Friends and Fitness Models

- Shama Chaudry we have only known each other a short time but you are truly amazing in your focus at the gym and in competitions.
- Robert Daniels before we ever knew each other a few years ago I witnessed your drive in the gym and many bodybuilding shows. What stands out the most is not your many trophies but your encouragement and kindness even when people came up to you when you clearly had your headphones on to focus on your own training.
- Bryan Eidem first I want to thank your for your friendship and encouragement through the years. Secondly for the many training sessions together as a coach and as a friend. Bryan without your introduction and training for the

International Natural Bodybuilding Association I would never have competed in shows myself.

Thank you to Cassandra Aaron for her time and the eye of an artist working with the Camera and Fitness Models, turning ideas into reality.

Last but not least a big thank you to my family, friends and training clients who have made transformations of their very own which has given me the dream and confidence to help even more people.

TABLE OF CONTENTS

Chapter 1. Introduction

When you get out of bed in the morning and start to get ready for work, do you avoid meeting your own gaze in the mirror?

Do you struggle to choose an outfit that flatters your body and doesn't make you feel bad about yourself?

Is it hard for you to make it up a flight of stairs without feeling winded or having to stop to rest?

If you answered "Yes" to any of these questions, you are not alone! As you may have already learned, the CDC estimates that more than 78 million American adults struggle with being overweight or obesity. Obesity has become something of an epidemic in this country and it is a problem that will not soon disappear.

Unfortunately, many people who are overweight or obese do not take accountability for themselves and for their problem. They blame the media for perpetuating unrealistic body image goals and they blame the fast food industry for their unhealthy habits. If you find yourself in a similar boat, it may be time for you to step up and face the reality of your situation.

Before you stop reading, thinking that I am just another fitness junkie who fat-shames people, consider this: I was once in your shoes! There was a time when I weighed more than 330 pounds so I know the struggles you are experiencing and I know how difficult it can be to make a change!

What I want you to know, however, is that change is possible, even if it is hard! Sometimes all you need is a little boost to get you moving in the right direction and that is exactly what I hope to provide with this book. It is my goal to help you start believing in yourself again – to help you see that a healthy future is possible and that you may already have the skills and tools you need to achieve it!

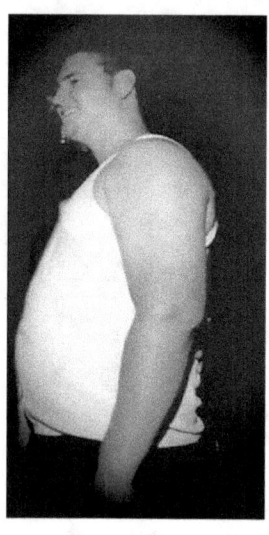

Believe me, I know what it feels like to be fat. I've been called every name in the book and I spent years feeling like I was worthless because I didn't look like the people I saw on TV. It was difficult for me to even care about eating healthy or exercising because I thought it would all be a wasted effort – I would never be fit.

When I finally took responsibility for myself and for my lifestyle, however, I discovered a strength I never knew I had. I found the courage I needed to look at myself in the mirror – and I mean REALLY look. What I saw was not just a person who was fat and unhappy. I was actually able to see the old me buried under pounds and pounds of fat. I realized that the old me (the me I wanted to be) was still in there and I had the power to bring him back!

The road was long and hard, but once I started to take myself and my goals seriously I began to lose weight. My clothes started to feel loose and I noticed that I didn't take up as much space when I sat in the driver's seat of my car. It did not take me as long to recover after climbing a flight of stairs and I was able to actually enjoy myself when my family went for a walk. I'm not saying it was easy, but I put in the work and it paid off!

Dropping more than 100 pounds of fat took time and more than a little bit of effort. Unfortunately, I was woefully uneducated about the basics of nutrition and fitness when I began my journey so I experienced a lot of hiccups along the way. The benefit for you is that I've already made the big mistakes so you don't have to!

In this book you will find a detailed summary of my experience to show you that I do indeed understand where you are coming from. I came to a point in my life where I simply couldn't stand to keep following the path I was walking and I committed myself to making a change. In reading this book you will learn the dangers of the modern American diet (like the one I was following for so many years) and the power of clean eating in transforming your eating habits and your life.

For me, the biggest changes happened when I altered my diet. I stopped eating fast food and processed food, focusing instead on lean proteins, fresh fruits and vegetables, and healthy fats. You have probably already heard of the Paleo diet but you may be skeptical about it since it seems so restrictive to people at first. Once you read about my experience with the diet, however, you may change your mind and decide to give it a shot! After you get used to it, the diet is really very easy to follow and you can still enjoy plenty of delicious (and healthy!) foods.

Improving my nutrition is what started the weight loss train rolling, but it really picked up speed when I started to exercise more regularly. Don't worry, I'm not going to tell you to start training for the marathon and I won't say that you have to spend two hours in the gym every day. I found that simply being more active and learning the basics of strength training was enough to boost my weight loss significantly while also helping me to gain lean muscle mass.

In addition to teaching you about healthy eating habits and weight lifting, I also want to help you set reachable goals for yourself. By following my advice in this book you will gain the skills you need to lose 100 pounds or more, but keep in mind that it will take time! If you set a goal for 100 pounds of weight loss in three months, or even six months, you may become discouraged when you do not reach that goal. I am not telling you that you should give up on your dreams or that you should not try your hardest – I am just saying that you need to set realistic expectations for yourself. When you reach those goals, then, you will be motivated to strive for the next milestone!

It is my hope that in reading this book you will come to realize that you have the power to change your life – you just need a little bit of direction and a push to get you started. By the time you finish this book you will have all of the tools you need to transform your life and your body.

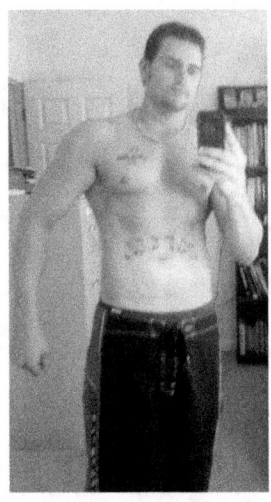

So, if you are ready to get up off the couch and start moving toward a better and brighter future, simply turn the page and keep reading! I guarantee you won't be disappointed!

Garry Bradley 300lbs to 200lbs

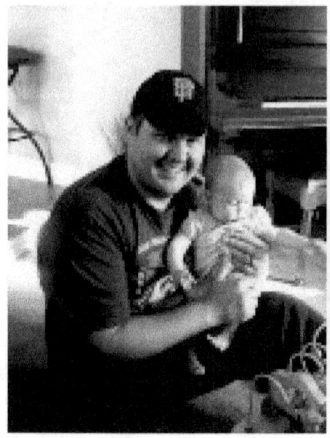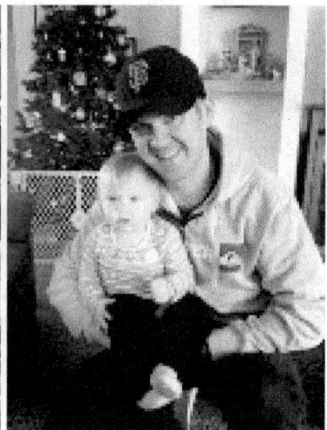

When our first child was born I wanted to take better care of myself so that I would be around for them, and be able to enjoy being active with them. I started by tracking my calorie intake and jogging a little. As the weight began to come off I took up cycling and fell in love with it. My starting weight was 300lbs. and 8 months later I was down to 200lbs. I didn't have to deny myself any food, if I wanted a snack food like ice cream I planned my meals for that day around it. My best advice is to find a system that works for you and stick with it. And if you have a bad day don't beat yourself up over it, just forgive yourself and start fresh tomorrow. It's not a race, it's a journey ~Garry Bradley

Chapter 2. My Story

Okay, so you already know a little bit about my story. I dropped more than 100 pounds simply by improving my eating habits and getting some healthy exercise. At this point, you may still be a little skeptical. After all, you've probably had the merits of "diet and exercise" drilled into your head for years like I had.

If you are willing to follow me for just a little bit longer, however, I want to give you the details of my story so you can understand exactly how I made my transformation and so you can see that you have the power to make the same changes in your own life.

The Day I Decided to Change

I come to you now, ten years after I decided to change my life, and I can say that I am a completely different person from who I was back then.

Well, that is not exactly what I mean. I weigh more than 100 pounds less than I used to but the biggest changes I experienced were not physical. Sure, I lost nearly 30% of my body weight in fat but what I gained is so much more important. I gained confidence in myself and came to view myself as a valuable, worthwhile person. I realized that I had the power to change my life within me all along, I simply had to activate it.

Before I get going into the details of how I changed my life I want to give you a little bit more insight into my life before

13

I decided to make the change. As you read this, you will probably draw some connections to your own life.

My Emotional Journey

One day about 10 years ago now I rolled out of bed at my usual time of 5:30 am. As was true of many mornings, I slowly wandered into the bathroom to start getting ready for work. I avoided meeting my own gaze in the mirror as long as I could until I absolutely had to look in order to make sure that my hair wasn't a mess.

When I met my own eyes in the mirror I experienced a rush of negative emotions. The person I saw looking back at me was not the same person that I felt inside. My face was large and round, my stomach protruded from my shirt, and I could barely see my toes if I looked down. As I picked apart myself in the mirror, a wave of pain and sadness washed over me as I recalled the events of the previous day.

My family owns a tree service and I had spent many years working for the company. Years of physical labor had helped me build a great deal of strength but my muscles were barely visible under the thick layers of fat I was carrying around. As my uncle drove the truck I found myself doing push-ups for fun in the back of the truck – I liked to challenge myself and somehow, being able to do 30 push-ups in a row made me feel as if my weight wasn't really *that* bad.

As I was doing my push-ups, I happened to overhear my uncle and my cousin (who was riding in the passenger seat) laughing over my belly – it was hanging out of my shirt and it touched the ground before my chest did as I did my push-ups. They didn't know that I had heard them, but their comments cut me pretty deep.

I am not the kind of person whose feelings are easily hurt but there was just something about the way they laughed that really got to me. I immediately became self-conscious not only about the way my belly hung low to the ground but also about the way my shirt stretched tight across my chest and the way my legs barely fit into my work pants. These feelings combined with the memories of people making fun of me for my weight and I came to a breaking point.

As I looked at myself in the mirror, experiencing all of these emotions anew, I began to take stock of myself. My feet hurt because I was starting to develop planter fasciitis. My knees and ankles were sore from the strain of supporting my body weight and my back was in knots as well. Lifting the hem of my shirt revealed a roadmap of stretch marks across my belly and sides, wrapping all the way around my back.

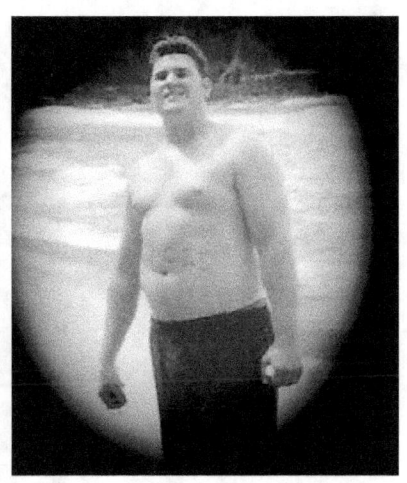

What really broke me down, however, was not just the image of my current self but the stark difference between the present and the past. As a child and a young man I spent a lot of time mountain biking and swimming. I loved to hike on the weekends and I never really had a problem with my weight until I hit my twenties – that is when my poor habits really caught up to me. After coming home from work I would sit down in front of the television with a bag of chips instead of going out with my friends or getting any exercise. It took a few years, but eventually I became so large that even the simplest forms of exercise became difficult for me.

Even now, 10 years after the fact, I still feel the pangs of hurt and disappointment that I felt when I overheard my cousin and my uncle. I may be 100 pounds lighter but I am still the same man and I shudder a little bit when I think of how much I let myself go and what might have happened had I not changed my life.

Find what motivates you! List out your motivating factors, have you suffered emotional pain or physical pain like I have? Do you have children or want children some day and want to set a good example and be healthy enough to run around with them.
Have you had an unwelcome health event that may have been an eye opener to you?

Let me share with you a quote from one of my favorite Authors and Pod-casters **Dan Miller**.

"Perhaps the unwelcome event you've encountered is just an opportunity to help you know how to stand up stronger."

List as many motivating factors as you can for when times get tough, start with 3 before you move on with this book and continue to add to this list for when it feels like it is getting tough.

Visit Link to download your free printable workbook

http://www.derekacox.com/killing-fat/

MY ROADMAP FOR TRANSFORMATION

As I have already told you, my journey to lose 100 pounds was not easy and it was most certainly not short. I didn't simply decide one day to lose weight and then immediately make it happen – it took weeks for me to learn the basics of nutrition and weight lifting and it took months for me to really get into the habit of maintaining healthy habits.

I don't want to discourage you into thinking that your hopes for weight loss are doomed – I just want you to understand that the journey will be long and hard. If you understand this going into it, you will be better able to overcome the challenges you face and to keep moving forward.

But you are probably wondering exactly what I did to lose weight and how you can achieve the same thing. Don't worry, I will give you all the details you need!

When I decided to buckle down and really change my life I took some time to really take stock of things. I printed out some pictures of my current self to remind me of where I was coming from as well as some pictures of my younger, fit self to use as inspiration for where I hoped to go. I also printed out pictures of the unhealthy foods and habits that had gotten me to this point and posted them on the refrigerator, inside my kitchen cabinets, anywhere I would see them and be reminded of my goals.

After doing a great deal of research I settled on the Paleo diet as my nutrition tool for weight loss. I had heard about the diet before but, if I'm being honest, I always scoffed a little bit at the idea of it. Cutting out all grains and dairy? Not eating things like beans and sugar? I thought a person had to be crazy to give up those foods. But I eventually came to realize that if I wanted to see big results I would have to make some big changes.

It took a few weeks for me to get the hang of it, but eventually it became second nature for me to follow the

Paleo diet. I found that I stopped missing processed foods and fast foods and I actually started to enjoy cooking for myself. I began craving healthy foods like fresh, crunchy salads and tender cuts of meat. I even found that I no longer craved sugary sodas and snacks!

The Paleo diet was definitely one of the biggest tools I used to achieve my weight loss goals but it was not the only one. In addition to improving my eating habits I also made changes to my lifestyle. I made an effort to be active every day, even if it was just a little bit. I took the stairs instead of the elevator; I parked my car a little bit further from the front door when I went grocery shopping; I spent 20 minutes of every morning walking around the block near my home. I really started to see results however, when I began lifting weights.

Before you start worrying about gym memberships, complicated exercises, and soreness from working out, let me stop you. Strength training is way simpler than many people make it out to be. You don't have to lift like a bodybuilder to gain muscle – in fact, you can perform just a few simple exercises two or three days a week to see huge results. It is really the combination of a healthy diet and regular exercise that helped me lose the 100 pounds.

You don't necessarily have to hire a personal trainer to start lifting, but I would recommend it. Personally, I signed up for a few sessions just to make sure that I learned the proper technique for various exercises. If you have never lifted before I would recommend at least one session with a trainer, just to get yourself started on the right foot.

After I learned the basics of weight lifting I started strength training two or three days a week for about 45 to 60 minutes. That is all the time it took for me to perform the key exercises that helped me to burn fat and build muscle. Later in this book I will walk you through the basics of weight training and help you create an exercise program that suits your needs.

Nutrition and exercise were the two key portions of a three-pronged attack. The third element in my transformative journey involved setting realistic goals and motivating myself to succeed. I started by making a dream board of all the things I hoped to do after I lost the weight and I used it to inspire me when things got tough. After walking you through the basics of nutrition and exercise I will teach you about setting SMART goals and give you some tips for staying motivated on your own journey.

ACTION STEP #2

Create your own dream board! Collect pictures, quotes, brochures, advertisements, anything that represents the end goal of your journey. Where do you see yourself at the end of your journey and what kind of things do you hope to do or achieve once you've reached it? Put all of the pictures together on a bulletin board and place it somewhere that you will see it every day. As you progress and start to accomplish small goals along the way you can add to the dream board.

Visit Link to download your free printable workbook

http://www.derekacox.com/killing-fat/

CHAPTER 3. THE POWER OF CLEAN EATING

Before I started my weight loss journey I was not at all concerned about healthy eating. I ate what I wanted, when I wanted it. Unhealthy eating habits are probably what caused my weight gain and my reluctance to give them up is what kept me from achieving my goals for so long.

If you have never heard the term "clean eating" before you may be a little nervous to learn about what it entails. Do not worry – I am not going to tell you that you have to count every calorie that passes your lips or that you can't eat anything but green salads and grilled chicken. The concept of clean eating is really very simple – the less altered the food is, the better. The goal is simply to eat wholesome, natural foods that have not been processed.

Before I get into the details about the dietary portion of my transformation program I want you to understand the dangers of your current eating habits. You may not realize it, but the eating habits you follow now could cut years off your life and increase your risk for some very serious diseases. In this chapter I will teach you about the risks of maintaining your current eating habits and walk you through the basics of clean eating.

Dangers of the Modern American Diet

According to the President's Council on Fitness, Sports & Nutrition, the average American diet exceeds the daily recommended levels for four different categories – sodium, saturated fats, refined grains, and added sugar. It is not just the adults that have unhealthy eating habits, either. It is estimated that empty calories from fats and added sugars account for up to 40% of total daily calorie intake for children between 2 and 18 years of age. Most of these empty calories come from things like soft drinks, desserts, whole milk, and pizza.

Many people have some level of understanding that fast food, processed foods, refined grains, and added sugars are bad but they do not understand how these foods correlate to some very real and very serious consequences. It is estimated that by the year 2030, more than half of American adults (that's about 115 million) will be obese. The statistics for children are not any better – adolescents that are overweight have a 70% chance of becoming overweight or obese adults.

The term "obesity" is defined as an excessively high amount of body fat in relation to lean body mass. One of the most common tools for determining obesity is BMI – or Body Mass Index. This is a measurement taken which correlates the height and weight of an individual along a numbered scale. The higher the person's weight is in comparison to his height, the higher his numerical BMI value. Values below 18.5 are considered underweight while values between 18.5 and 24.9

are considered normal. Values between 25 and 29.9 are overweight and values above 30 are obese.

Though a number of factors can contribute to a person becoming overweight or obese, diet is the main factor. According to the Pritikin Longevity Center and Spa, the things that Americans eat are more dangerous to our health than any other factor. While it may be true that modern Americans live longer in general, diseases caused by obesity can take years off of a person's life.

You probably already know that obesity is bad for your health, but have you actually taken the time to learn the details? How exactly does obesity affect your lifespan and what kind of diseases are you putting yourself at risk for by maintaining your current weight?

<u>Below you will find a list of diseases or conditions that are directly related to or impacted by obesity</u>:

High Blood Pressure – Also known as hypertension, high blood pressure can lead to excess pressure in the arteries and it can be damaging to the body in many ways.

Coronary Heart Disease – When your BMI increases, so does the risk for CHD. This is a condition where a waxy buildup (called plaque) forms inside your arteries, blocking blood flow (and thus oxygen deliver) to the heart. If the heart cannot pump enough blood, the body will go into heart failure and this can be fatal.

Stroke – The buildup of plaque in your arteries doesn't just impair blood flow to the heart – it also impacts the delivery of oxygen to other parts of the body, especially the brain.

When an area of plaque ruptures it causes a blood clot to form and if the clot blocks oxygen and blood flow to the brain it can cause a stroke.

Type 2 Diabetes – This disease occurs when blood sugar levels in the body are too high. This can be the result of an insufficient production or use of insulin, or it can be caused by eating high-glycemic foods. If your blood sugar remains too high for too long, the body becomes resistant to the effects of insulin and that causes Type 2 diabetes.

High Cholesterol – There are two types of cholesterol: high-density lipoprotein (HDL) or "good" cholesterol, and low-density lipoprotein (LDL) or "bad" cholesterol. High LDL levels can increase the risk for coronary heart disease as well as a number of other conditions.

Metabolic Syndrome – Not a singular disease but a group of risk factors that increases the risk for heart disease and other conditions, metabolic syndrome is defined by the occurrence of three or more of the following factors:

- Large waistline
- Higher than normal triglyceride levels
- Lower than normal HDL levels
- Higher than normal blood pressure
- Higher than normal blood sugar levels

Osteoarthritis – The more extra weight you are carrying, the more quickly the protective tissues in your joints will be worn down. For people who are overweight or obese, osteoarthritis in the back as well as the knees, hips, and ankles is common.

Cancer – Being overweight or obese can significantly increase your risk for certain types of cancer including breast cancer, colon cancer, gallbladder cancer, and endometrial cancer.

Sleep Apnea – This is a condition in which a person experiences one or more pauses in breathing during sleep. People who have a high BMI tend to have more fat stored in the neck area which can place pressure on the airway during sleep, causing the airway to collapse.

Gallstones – These are small, hard, stone-like formations primarily made up of cholesterol which can form in the gallbladder. Gallstones are common in people who are overweight or obese and they can cause severe back and stomach pain.

After reading this information you cannot deny that the modern American diet is very unhealthy. But what is it about the modern American diet that is so bad? According to research conducted in 2010, there are nearly a dozen components of the modern American diet which can be damaging to the human body. These factors include:

- Low in fruits
- Low in vegetables
- Low in nuts and seeds
- Low in whole grains
- Low in fiber
- Low in omega-3 fatty acids
- Low in polyunsaturated fatty acids
- High in sodium
- High in trans fats

- High in sugar-sweetened beverages
- High in processed meats

After reading this list, take a moment to think about your own diet. How many of these components play a key role in your own diet? If you are honest with yourself you may be forced to admit that most or all of these things are true for you. Fortunately, you can boost your health and gain back some of your lost years by improving your eating habits.

What is Clean Eating?

The term "clean eating" is not meant to reference any particular diet. Rather, it is a term used to describe a certain dietary philosophy – the idea that wholesome, natural foods with minimal processing or alteration are the best foods to consume. Many of the most popular diets that are currently in existence adhere to this general philosophy, even if the details of the specific diet vary.

To help you get an idea what clean eating looks like, consider the seven rules of clean eating listed below:

1. Choose whole, natural, and unprocessed foods over foods that have been processed or otherwise altered by man (generally, you should avoid foods that come in a box, can, or bag – some exceptions are for whole fruits and vegetables).

2. Always choose unrefined over refined foods (choose whole grains and natural sweeteners over refined grains and sugars).

3. Balance each meal with protein, carbohydrate, and fat (try to include some protein in each meal and don't go overboard on carbohydrates).

4. Limit your intake of fat, salt, and sugar (focus on healthy fats and flavor your foods with natural herbs and spices instead of salt).

5. Eat up to six small meals per day instead or two or three large meals (breaking up your meals over the course of the day will keep your metabolism and your energy up – it may also help to prevent snacking and overeating at meals).

6. Avoid drinking your calories when possible (avoid high-calorie beverages especially sugary sodas, alcoholic beverages, and coffee drinks – drink plenty of water and herbal tea).

7. Incorporate physical exercise into your daily routine (get moving in any way you can).

If you follow these seven simple rules you will not need to worry about detailed lists of foods you should and should not be eating. Before you eat something, simply ask yourself, "Has this food been changed in any way?" If the food has been processed, refined, artificially flavored, sweetened, or changed in any unnatural way, it is best avoided.

ACTION STEP #3

Take stock of your current eating habits. Now that you understand what clean eating is you should have a better idea of how your current eating habits might be negatively affecting your health. Keep track of all of the foods you eat over the course of one 24-hour period and then take a look at it to see just how many unhealthy foods you are eating on a regular basis. You may also want to clean out your kitchen and pantry, removing unhealthy foods and foods that trigger unhealthy habits.

Chapter 4. The Paleo Diet for Weight Loss

In the last chapter I introduced you to the concept of clean eating. This is a great place to start when you first begin your journey to transformation. After just a few days of avoiding processed foods and sugary beverages you may start to feel a difference in your energy levels and in your digestion. The longer you adhere to the principles of clean eating, the better you will feel!

After just a few weeks of clean eating myself I lost several pounds and I found that I experienced some other benefits as well. I was sleeping better, I was less tired during the day, I didn't get sugar cravings, and my digestion became more regular. Though I loved the changes I was experiencing with clean eating in general, I wondered what would happen if I took things one step further. So, I did the research and I decided to try the Paleo diet.

What is the Paleo Diet?

The Paleo diet is based on the way our ancestors lived, a very primitive hunter-gatherer lifestyles. Everything that humans ate where either caught and killed via hunting and fishing or gathered from the earth. The majority of the diet for humans consisted of meat, fruits, vegetables, nuts, and seeds.

The modern Paleo diet is loosely based on the dietary habits of our ancestors. The diet includes only those foods which can be safely consumed without any sort of processing –

this excludes dairy products (which are typically pasteurized) as well as grains and legumes. The modern Paleo diet also excludes all sugars except natural sweeteners (like honey and maple syrup) as well as soy products and hydrogenated oils. The focus for the modern Paleo diet is on fresh produce, lean meats and seafood, healthy oils, nuts, and seeds.

HISTORY OF THE PALEO DIET

The true Paleo diet is thousands of years old, but the modern interpretation of the diet has only been popularized within the last century or so. The first use of the term "Paleo Diet" was made by gastroenterologist Walter L. Voegtlin in his 1975 book, *The Stone Age Diet*. In this book, Voegtlin wrote that humans are natural carnivorous beings.

Voegtlin suggests that our bodies are naturally inclined to accept and even thrive on a Paleolithic-style diet. Voegtlin's claims did not earn him much notice during the 1970s but several researchers and health experts published additional works throughout the 80s and 90s which brought the Paleo diet into the mainstream. Today, the Paleo diet is one of the most popular diets among celebrities, trainers, and fitness experts.

BENEFITS OF THE PALEO DIET

The benefits of the Paleo diet overlap with the benefits of clean eating since they are founded on the same basic principles. The Paleo diet takes things a little bit further, however, by excluding all foods that are the result of agriculture or industry. This diet may take some getting used to but once you get into the habit you will experience a wide variety of different benefits.

<u>Some of the biggest health benefits the Paleo diet can provide include the following</u>:

Balanced blood sugar levels. The Paleo diet is naturally low-carb because it excludes grains and dairy products. This diet is also naturally low-glycemic as well.

Relief from food sensitivities. It is estimated that 1 in 100 people have Celiac disease (an autoimmune disease triggered by gluten) and as many as 15 million Americans suffer from food allergies. The Paleo diet is naturally gluten- and dairy-free, plus it is free from other common allergens like corn, wheat, and soy.

Lean muscle mass. The Paleo diet is naturally low in calories and high in protein which will help you to build a leaner physique.

Feel full longer with less snacking. Because the Paleo diet is focused on fresh, wholesome foods you may experience reduced food cravings. Eating whole foods like lean proteins and complex carbohydrates will also help to keep you feeling full for longer, helping you to avoid snacking.

No calorie counting required. The Paleo diet is more of a lifestyle choice than a fad diet and calorie counting is not a major part of the diet. If you are trying to lose weight you may want to keep an eye on your calorie consumption but calorie restriction is not part of the Paleo diet.

Reduced risk for chronic disease. As you already know, poor eating habits can greatly increase your risk for serious diseases like cancer, heart disease, and Type 2 diabetes. Improving your eating habits by following the Paleo diet will greatly improve your health and reduce your risk for disease.

Improved sleep habits. Many people who are overweight or obese report sleep problems such as insomnia or sleep apnea. When you switch to the Paleo diet you may experience relief from these problems – you may fall asleep more quickly and stay asleep through the night. You will also feel more rested and energized in the morning.

Detoxification from chemicals and processed foods. The Paleo diet is focused on all-natural foods so you may experience the detoxification benefits of ridding your body of synthetic chemicals and food additives.

Better overall nutrition and energy. The Paleo diet is naturally focused on healthy foods so it will boost your nutrition significantly. When you stop eating processed carbohydrates and start focusing on wholesome nutrition you will experience increased energy levels and a more regulated metabolism.

Healthy weight loss. For many people, switching to the Paleo diet is about weight loss. While this diet is not specifically intended for weight loss, improving your nutrition and cutting out processed foods and refined sugars can help you to lose weight naturally.

Every person's body responds differently to the Paleo diet so you may find that you experience some or all of these benefits. Remember, the longer you follow the diet and the more dedicated you are to the principles of clean eating, the more benefits you will receive.

SWITCHING TO THE PALEO DIET

For many people, the Paleo diet is drastically different from their typical eating habits. This being the case, it can take some time to get used to the new diet. One of the first things you'll need to do is familiarize yourself with the foods that are and are not included in the diet. Once you have an understanding of the Paleo diet food list you will be able to make simple changes to your diet over time to transition yourself onto the Paleo diet.

PALEO DIET FOOD LISTS

The Paleo diet may seem restrictive at first but the more you look at the food lists the more you will realize that you still have plenty of options. As a reminder, the main food groups allowed on the Paleo diet are lean meats and eggs, fish and seafood, nuts and seeds, fresh fruits and vegetables, and healthy fats and oils. To give you a better idea of what you will and will not be eating on the Paleo diet, consider the food lists on the following page:

Foods to Eat Freely

Protein Options:

- Eggs
- Chicken
- Turkey
- Duck
- Beef*
- Pork
- Veal*
- Lamb*
- Game Meat
- Sausage*
- Shrimp
- Crab
- Lobster
- Mussels
- Scallops
- Fish

Fresh Fruits and Vegetables

- Acorn Squash*
- Apples
- Apricots
- Asparagus
- Artichoke
- Arugula
- Banana
- Beets
- Bell Peppers
- Bok Choy
- Blackberries
- Blueberries
- Broccoli
- Brussels Sprouts
- Butternut Squash*
- Cabbage
- Carrots
- Cantaloupe
- Cauliflower
- Celery
- Cherries
- Cranberries
- Cucumber
- Dates
- Eggplant
- Fennel

- Figs
- Grapes
- Grapefruit
- Greens
- Green Beans
- Green Onion
- Guava
- Honeydew
- Kale
- Kohlrabi
- Kiwi
- Lemon
- Lettuce
- Lime
- Leeks
- Mango
- Mushrooms
- Nectarines
- Onions
- Papaya
- Parsnips
- Peaches
- Pears
- Pineapple
- Plums
- Pomegranate
- Pumpkin
- Raspberries
- Rutabaga
- Snow Peas
- Spaghetti Squash
- Spinach
- Strawberries
- Snap Peas
- Sweet Potato*
- Tomatoes
- Turnips
- Watercress
- Watermelon
- Zucchini

Healthy Fats and Oils

- Almonds
- Almond Butter
- Avocado
- Avocado Oil
- Brazil Nuts
- Cashews
- Chestnuts
- Chia Seeds
- Clarified Butter
- Coconut Milk
- Coconut Oil
- Flaxseeds
- Flaxseed Oil
- Hazelnuts

- Hemp Seeds
- Macadamia Nuts
- Olives
- Olive Oil
- Pecans
- Pine Nuts
- Pistachios
- Pumpkin Seeds
- Sesame Oil
- Sesame Seeds
- Sunflower Seeds
- Tallow
- Walnuts
- Walnut Oil

Pantry Staples and Other Foods

- Almond Flour
- Almond Milk
- Cider Vinegar
- Arrowroot Powder
- Balsamic Vinegar
- Broths and Stocks
- Cocoa Powder (Unsweetened)
- Coconut Aminos
- Coconut Flour
- Coconut Milk
- Coconut Sugar*
- Dark Chocolate*
- Fresh Herbs
- Fruit Juice*
- Ground Spices
- Honey (Raw)*
- Maple Syrup*
- Stevia Leaf
- Tapioca Flour
- Tapioca Starch
- Vanilla Extract

*These are foods which should be enjoyed in moderation due to calorie, fat, or sugar content. Be careful about how many cured meats you eat as well (like bacon) because they are high in nitrates and sodium.

Foods to Avoid Completely

Grains, Beans and Legumes

- All-Purpose Flour
- Amaranth
- Baking Mix
- Black Beans
- Buckwheat
- Cake Flour
- Corn
- Couscous
- Garbanzo Beans
- Kidney Beans
- Lentils
- Millet
- Oats
- Pastry Flour
- Peanuts
- Peanut Butter
- Pinto Beans
- Quinoa
- Rice
- Rye
- Semolina
- Sorghum
- Soybeans
- Spelt
- Wheat
- White Beans

Dairy Products

- Buttermilk
- Cheese
- Coffee Creamer
- Cottage Cheese
- Cream Cheese
- Frozen Yogurt
- Half n' Half
- Heavy Cream
- Ice Cream
- Kefir
- Milk
- Whipped Cream
- Yogurt

Pantry Staples and Other Foods

- Alcohol
- Artificial Sweeteners
- Bread
- Brown Sugar
- Candy
- Chocolate (Sweetened)
- Corn Syrup
- Cornstarch
- Granulated Sugar
- Energy Drinks
- Fast Food
- Frozen Dinners
- Granola Bars
- Pasta
- Pizza
- Processed Foods
- Sweetened Drinks
- Soy Sauce

TIPS FOR TRANSITIONING

Now that you know what foods you will and will not be eating on the Paleo diet you are ready to start making the transition. If your current diet is very heavily focused on processed foods and fast food, you may need to make some simple changes to your diet over time instead of making the switch all at once.

Many people who switch to the Paleo diet all at once experience some negative side effects similar to withdrawal. These symptoms may include headaches, fatigue, and irritability among others and they are generally caused by withdrawal from refined carbohydrates and sugar. In most cases, withdrawal symptoms go away within a week or so as long as you keep sticking to the Paleo diet.

If you are worried about withdrawal symptoms or you simply want to make the transition more slowly, here are a few tips to try:

- **Start increasing your daily consumption of fresh fruits and vegetables**. Try adding a banana to your morning meal or make a fruit and vegetable smoothie for an afternoon snack.
- **Try to replace fatty and processed meats with leaner options**. Instead of using ground beef to make hamburgers, try ground turkey or chicken. Start eating more fish and poultry products and switch over to grass-fed red meats.
- **Swap out hydrogenated and vegetable oils for healthy oils**. Choose olive oil or coconut oil for cooking over vegetable oil and canola oil.
- **Start decreasing your consumption of grains slowly**. You can try going from two pieces of toast in the morning to one slice or swap in a baked sweet potato instead of rice at dinner.
- **Decrease your use of refined sugar and start using natural sweeteners**. Try out some recipes using honey or maple syrup as the sweetener and stop using sugar or artificial sweeteners in your morning coffee.
- **Try to balance your consumption of protein, carbohydrates, and fat**. Make an effort to include protein in every meal and eat plenty of fresh fruits and vegetables as well.

Feel free to take as long as you need to transition onto the Paleo diet. Your first priority should be to learn and implement the principles of clean eating. Once you have that down you can then make the additional changes needed to switch over to the Paleo diet. To help you get started with the diet you will find some Paleo recipes and sample meal plans at the end of this book.

ACTION STEP #4

Stock your kitchen with healthy, Paleo-friendly foods! Now that you understand the basics of the Paleo diet and have received detailed food lists for what you should and should not be eating, you have the resources you need to restock your kitchen and pantry with Paleo-friendly foods. Refer to the food lists above and head to the grocery store to stock up – be sure to eat something before you go because grocery shopping on an empty stomach often leads to impulse buys. Once you've stocked your Paleo kitchen you can take advantage of the recipes and meal plans provided at the end of this book!

CHAPTER 5. WEIGHT LIFTING FOR BODY TRANSFORMATION

Committing to a workout plan is an essential part of your transformation journey. You do not necessarily need to become obsessive about it but you do need to be intentional. Aim for at least two workouts per week, ideally three or four. Your workouts do not have to be very long (you can perform an effective strength training session in under an hour) but you should be prepared to expend a moderate amount of energy at a minimum throughout the entire workout in order to achieve the maximum result.

In this chapter you will learn the basics of bodybuilding as well as some tips for creating an effective workout plan. Don't worry – I do not expect you to spend two hours a day in the gym and I don't expect you to have washboard abs after just a few months. The actual definition of bodybuilding might surprise you, especially if you are familiar with famous bodybuilders like Arnold Schwarzenegger. You will also learn the benefits of weight lifting in this chapter as well as the proper form for some of the most important strength training exercises to build your workout plan around.

WHAT IS BODYBUILDING?

Despite what you may think, bodybuilding doesn't have to mean bulging muscles and popping veins. A bodybuilder is simply someone who wants to build a better body. That's right – you can become a bodybuilder! Though the term bodybuilder is most commonly applied to muscle heads like Lou Ferrigno and Tom Platz, there are many different ways to interpret the word. I am a firm believer in the idea that anyone who takes steps to improve their fitness and to build a better body is a bodybuilder.

You may or may not agree with me on this point but what I really want you to think about is the importance of incorporating strength training into your workout plan. While cardiovascular exercise is a great way to burn calories, it is not the only path to fitness. The truth of the matter is that muscle burns more calories than fat so, if you can build muscle while losing weight your body will naturally burn additional calories without any extra effort on your part. That sounds pretty good, doesn't it?

BENEFITS OF WEIGHT LIFTING

While strength training doesn't have the same cardiovascular benefits as running or other cardio exercises, it does give your heart a bit of a workout. The main benefits of weight lifting, however, actually occur after you have finished your workout. Here are some of the benefits that have been associated with strength training:

Increased strength, power, and endurance. The more you use your muscles, the stronger you become. Not only does this apply to future workouts, but it will enhance your ability to fulfill everyday tasks with greater ease as well.

Improved flexibility. Working your muscles through their full range of motion will help you to improve your flexibility.

Enhanced flexibility has been associated with a reduced risk for injury, especially things like pulled muscles and back pain.

Better body composition. If you are trying to lose weight, your efforts will probably be focused on shedding fat. The more lean muscle you have, the higher your metabolism which means increased calorie burn and more fat lost.

Improved posture. Strengthening your muscles will not just make you look and feel better, but it will improve your posture as well. This can help to alleviate common issues like back pain and stiff neck.

Protects bone health and strength. Adding strength training to your workout plan can help to stop or even reverse bone loss. Stronger muscles mean stronger bones!

Maintained weight loss. When you do the work to lose weight and shed fat, you want to know that your results will stick. If you incorporate strength training into your workout plan your body will burn more calories on a daily basis (in addition to calories burned during exercise) to help you maintain a healthy weight.

Improved mood. The benefits of strength training are not just physical – they are psychological as well! Studies have shown that strength training boosts endorphin production, helping you to feel better – you may sleep better as well!

These are just a few of the many benefits associated with strength training. Do you believe me now when I say that it is an important part of any workout plan?

CREATING A WORKOUT PLAN

There are countless different workout plans out there, but many of them seem to be designed for people who are already in shape. For example, popular fitness programs like P90X and Insanity require a certain degree of cardiovascular fitness just to make it through the workout. If you want to try these programs for yourself you are more than welcome, but I don't want you to become discouraged if you find yourself struggling. I would rather you take it easy and start with something simple and build on it than start a program that is too difficult and end up quitting.

What I want you to come away from this chapter knowing is that workouts do not have to be complicated! The most important thing is that you are moving and engaging your muscles – how you make that happen is up to you. If you are afraid of weight lifting because you have never tried it before, don't be nervous! I will give you the information you need to learn the basic movements that you can then use to build a custom workout plan for yourself.

Basic Weight Lifting Exercises

If you have never belonged to a gym before you might be overwhelmed the first time you set foot in one. Looking around at all of the machines and the rows upon rows of free weights you may have no idea where to begin. If you are completely new to weight lifting, the machines are not a bad place to start. Most gyms offer free consultations and a tour of the facilities during which you can ask questions or ask for a demonstration for using the different machines. Many gyms organize their machines in groups based on the muscles they work so it is easy to divide your weekly workouts accordingly.

For those who may have some weight lifting experience, or if you simply prefer to use free weights there are five main exercises you should know. Using these exercises you can work all of the main muscle groups in your body during a single 45- to 60-minute workout. Once you have mastered these exercises you can add supplementary exercises to work specific muscles or muscle groups.

The five most basic weight lifting exercises are as follows:

Deadlift

The name of this exercise may sound daunting but it is actually fairly simple to master and it is one of the most effective exercises as well since it works all of the major muscles in the body. This exercise is performed standing with feet shoulder-width apart, a loaded barbell on the floor in front of you. Bend at the knees, preserving the natural arch of your back, and grip the barbell with both hands. Then, use your glutes and quads to explode upward, keeping your weight in your heels as you stand up straight. Return to the starting position for the next repetition.

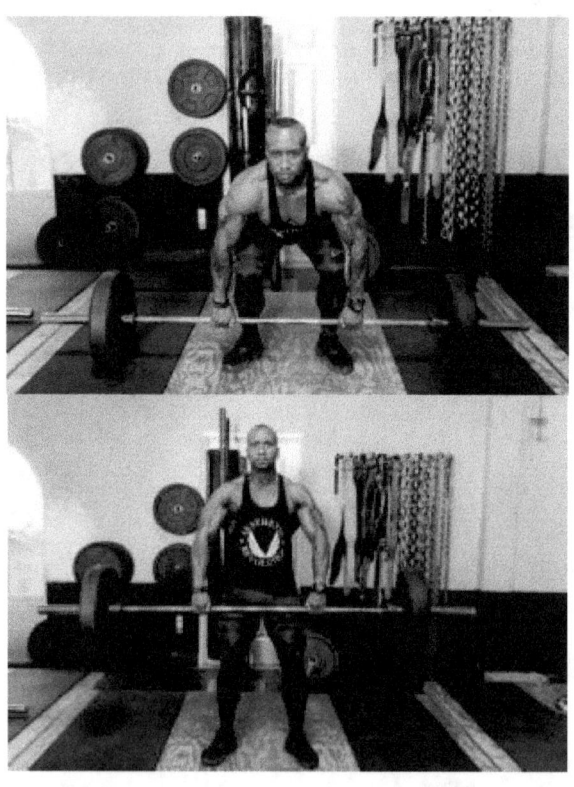

Squat

The squat is by far the best exercise for lower-body training. Not only does it work all of the major muscle groups in your body but it gives you a bit of cardiovascular exercise as well by boosting your heart rate. To perform this exercise, hold a barbell on your shoulders with a wide hand grip, standing with your feet slightly wider than shoulder-width apart. Bend at the knees, thrusting your hips back to preserve the natural arch of your back and keeping your knees from going past your toes, and lower yourself until your thighs are parallel to the ground. Drive your weight back into your heels to return to the starting position for one repetition.

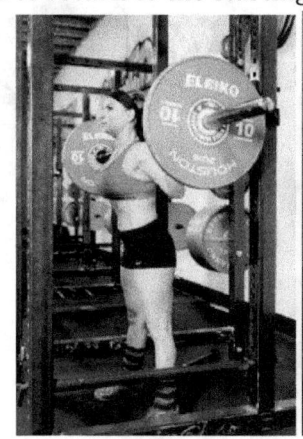 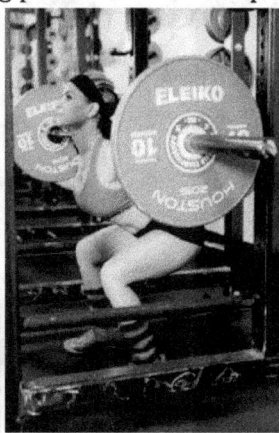

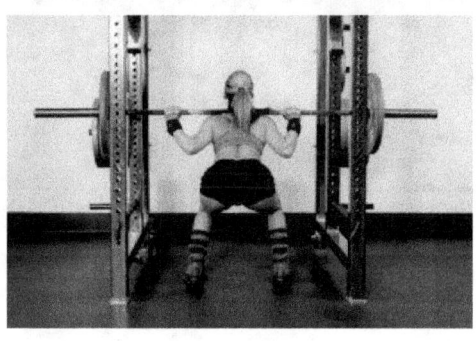

Push-Up – It may surprise you to see this exercise on the list but push-ups are actually a great exercise. Not only do they help to build upper body strength but they will work your core as well as your legs. There are many different variations on the push-up that you can try as you build strength to make things more challenging. To perform a push-up with good form start with your hands slightly more than shoulder-width apart, making a straight line with your body. Slowly lower your chest to the ground (be careful not to bend at the waist) then raise yourself back up for one repetition.

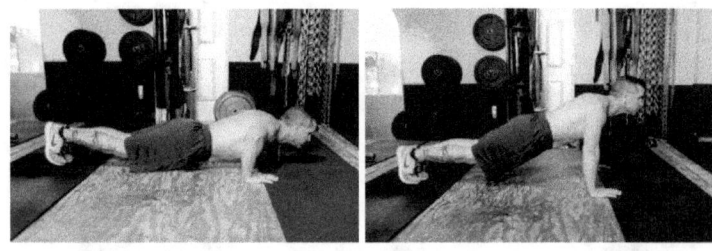

Push-Up Modified – If you can't do a full push-up modify the position by doing an **Incline push-up** by pressing off a bench or table instead of letting your knees touch the floor to keep your core involved in stabilizing you.

Bench Press - The Bench Press is a compound exercise. It works your chest, shoulders, triceps and a few other stabilizing muscles. It's the most effective exercise to gain upper-body strength and muscle. To start you will be lying on the bench with your feet on the floor. Your grip should be a little wider then shoulder width, un-rack the bar with straight arms lower the bar to your mid-chest and press it back up making sure to keep your feet plated and your butt on the bench.

Warning- Make sure to have someone Spot you while doing a Bench Press or use a chest press machine at the gym because if you push yourself to failure you may miss the re-rack and become stuck under the weight.

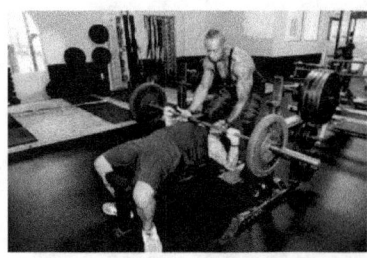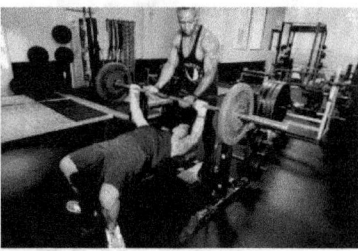

Overhead Press - The Overhead Press is the one of the best exercises for building strong and healthy shoulders. The overhead press is a full body, compound exercise that you use your shoulders and arms to press the weight over your head while your legs, lower back and abs stabilize you. Start by standing with the bar on your shoulders grip should be about shoulder width apart. Press the bar over your head until your arms are fully extended and shrug your shoulders at the top. Keep your core tight and legs steady. Lower the bar to your shoulders and repeat.

Make sure you start with a light weight and press slowly to ensure your balance with weight overhead.

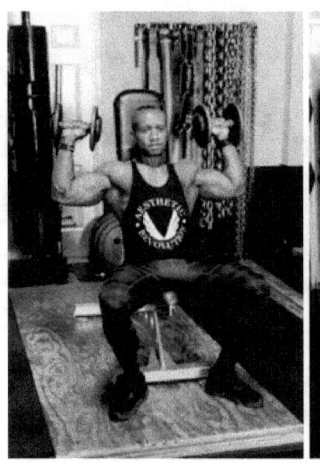 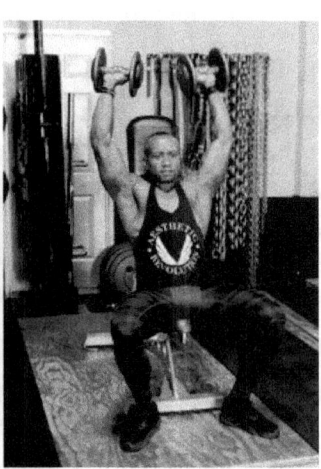

Pull-Up – The pull-up is one of the best exercises to work the muscles in your upper back and shoulders. Performing a pull-up with good form requires you to maintain tension throughout the entire body which makes it a full-body exercise. There are different variations on the pull-up that you can try to work different muscles in your upper body. To perform a pull-up correctly, grip the bar a little more than shoulder-width apart, your palms facing away from you. Engage your core and pull yourself up so your chin comes up over the bar. Slowly lower yourself back down until your arms are fully extended then repeat for as many repetitions as you can.

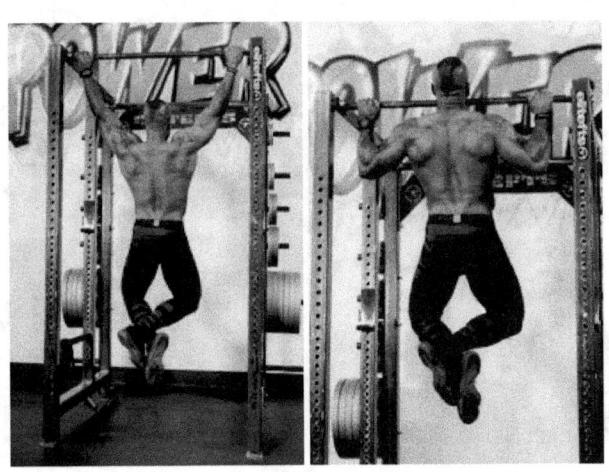

Lat Pulldown – If a Pull up is still to difficult you can perform Lat pulldowns to strengthen your muscles working your way up to completing the pull-up. The pulldown usually uses a weight machine with a seat and brace for the thighs. The starting position involves sitting at the machine with the thighs braced, back straight and feet flat on the floor. The arms are held overhead at full extension, holding a bar connected to the weight stack. The movement is performed by pulling the elbows down and back, lowering the bar to the neck, and completed by returning to the starting position.

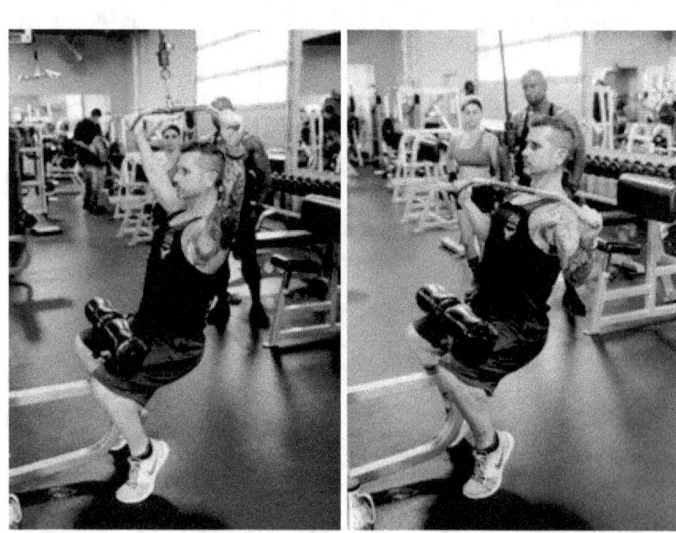

Barbell Row - The Barbell Row is a full body, compound exercise that will work your upper-back, lower back, hips and arms. They build a strong, muscular back and bigger arms. Barbell Rows are one of the most effective exercises you can do to increase your Squat, Bench Press and Deadlift.

Start with the bar on the floor. Bend over and grab the bar with your palms facing down. Pull the bar against your lower chest while keeping your torso horizontal. Keep your lower back neutral not letting it round or you could injure it. To finish the Rep you will return the bar to the floor.

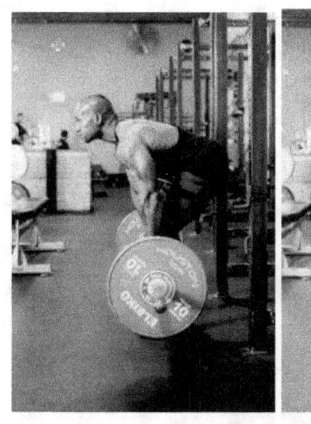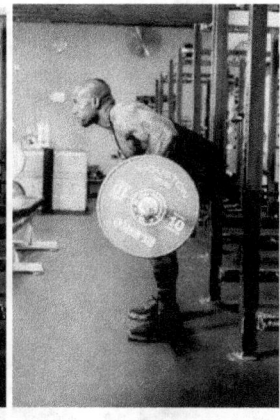

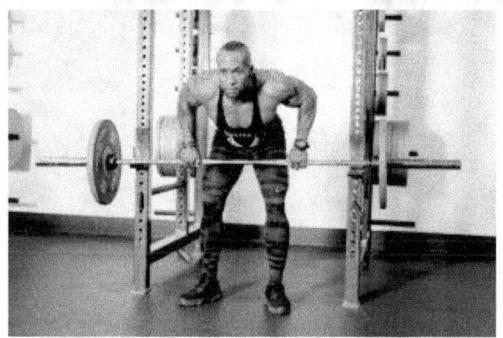

Lunge – There are many different ways to do lunges but they all work the muscles in your lower body – your glutes, hamstrings, quads, and even your calves. The most effective form of the lunge is the side lunge and, to get started, you simply stand with your feet hip-width apart. Step out to the side with your right foot as wide as you can, keeping both feet pointed forward. Shift your weight into your right foot, pushing the hips back and bending the knee. Lunge until your shinbone is perpendicular to the floor and your knee is right over your toe. Push off your right foot firmly and return to the starting position then repeat on the opposite side.

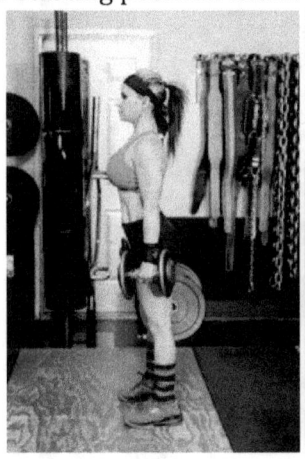
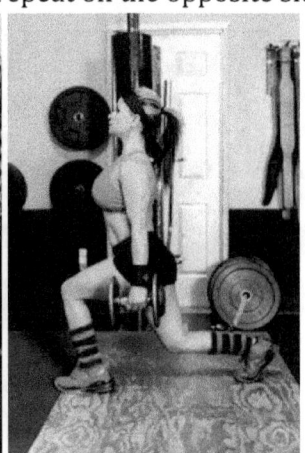

In addition to these exercises there are some other basic moves you may want to familiarize yourself with. The bench press, for example, is a great exercise for working your chest muscles – it also works your shoulders and triceps. To perform this exercise you lie flat on a bench, lowering the barbell to your chest and then raising it straight back up – this is one repetition. Another good exercise to learn is the barbell row – this is similar to the deadlift except you keep your back bent and use your arms to lift the barbell to your chest, working your upper and lower back as well as your hips and arms.

Once you have learned how to perform the deadlift, squat, bench press and barbell row you only need to learn one more exercise to follow the popular StrongLifts 5x5 program. The final exercise in this program is the overhead press. This exercise is performed standing up while holding a barbell to your chest. You use your shoulders and arms to press the weight over your head, using your legs and core strength to balance yourself.

The StrongLifts 5x5 program is a great example of a simple workout plan for beginners. All you need is five simple exercises and you only need to perform the workouts three days per week – just make sure you leave at least one day of rest in between your workouts.

On the following page you will find an example workout plan for this program:

Week 1 Workout Plan		
Workout 1	**Workout 2**	**Workout 3**
Squat 5x5	Squat 5x5	Squat 5x5
Overhead Press 5x5	Bench Press 5x5	Overhead Press 5x5
Deadlift 1x5	Barbell Row 5x5	Deadlift 1x5

Week 2 Workout Plan		
Workout 1	**Workout 2**	**Workout 3**
Squat 5x5	Squat 5x5	Squat 5x5
Bench Press 5x5	Overhead Press 5x5	Bench Press 5x5
Barbell Row 5x5	Deadlift 1x5	Barbell Row 5x5

Following the StrongLifts 5x5 program you would perform the exercises indicated on the chart above for each workout. The 5x5 simply means that you perform five sets of five repetitions with the same amount of weight. The goal is to gain enough strength to perform all five sets with good form. Once you are able to do so for all five sets, you increase the weight by 5 pounds for your next workout.

The StrongLifts 5x5 program is just an example of a workout plan that is good for beginners. If you like, you can find another program that suits your needs or you can build a program yourself.

Tips for Building a Workout Plan

Once you learn the proper form for the five basic exercises you have the skills necessary to build your own custom workout plan. Remember, you should build your workout plan around the five main exercises mentioned in the last section to ensure that you work out all of the major muscle groups in your body – you can then add additional exercises if you want to work smaller muscles like the biceps, triceps, or calves.

When building a workout plan you need to think about your goals in order to determine the ideal number of repetitions for each exercise. A repetition is simply the name given to a single performance of one exercise. A set is a group of repetitions. If you want to improve general fitness and tone your muscles, perform 10 to 15 repetitions of each exercise per set. If you want to build muscle and increase strength, perform 6 to 8 repetitions in each set.

The higher the number of repetitions, the lower the weight should be. This means that if your maximum weight for deadlifting is 100 pounds and you want to aim for fitness and toned muscles, you may want to decrease the weight to 80 or 90 pounds for 15 repetitions per set. If you are trying to build muscle and increase strength, use the maximum amount of weight at which you can safely perform 6 to 8 repetitions with good form.

While strength training is the key to building muscle and strength, you should also try to work some cardiovascular activity into your rotation. Cardiovascular activity doesn't have to mean running – if walking is as much as you can handle, that is completely fine. Another option for cardio is swimming, biking, or dancing. If you have trouble motivating yourself to be more active, try joining a Zumba class or another group fitness class that will keep you accountable while also being fun.

As you build your workout plan, don't be afraid to start small. Three days of exercise a week (two days of lifting and one day of cardio) is a good place to start. As you lose weight and become fitter you can add an additional workout to your week or simply extend the length of your workouts. Just pick a plan that you can stick to and focus on doing the exercises correctly and with good form.

ACTION STEP #4

Commit to exercising three times per week. It is up to you how you want to structure your exercise plan but a good place to start is with three workouts per week, at least two of those workouts including strength training exercises. If you are new to exercise you may want to start small with three 30-minute walks per week until your cardiovascular fitness improves a little bit. Once you are able to handle longer periods of exercise you can start to work in more rigorous cardio sessions as well as strength training sessions.

Chapter 6. Taking Back Control of Your Life

At this point you have the information and the tools you need to be successful in your weight loss journey. But how do you actually get started? If you do not set goals for yourself before you start your journey, how will you know when you've achieved success? Having specific and reachable goals in mind will help you to motivate yourself to keep going – the more goals you meet and the more progress you make, the more motivated you will be!

When I first started improving my diet and exercising on a regular basis I had one goal in mind: lose weight. I eventually came to realize, however, that this goal wasn't quite specific enough. How much weight did I want to lose? Did I want to lose a certain number of pounds or did I want to see inches lost from certain areas? Once I took the time to really think about the direction I wanted to go in I was able to set some specific goals and I kept track of my progress toward those goals throughout the process.

In this chapter I will teach you how to set SMART goals for yourself. The key is to set multiple progressive goals so that once you reach a milestone, you have the next milestone lined up.

Setting SMART Goals

The term SMART is an acronym which stands for Specific, Measurable, Attainable, Realistic, and Timely. This acronym is a useful guide to keep in mind when setting goals for yourself. It is not enough to simply say that you want to lose weight – you need to set a timeline and an end goal for yourself as well as multiple smaller goals along the way. In addition to setting these goals, you also need to keep track of your progress in measurable ways. To help you understand how this works, consider the SMART acronym:

Specific – A specific goal answers the questions Who, What, When, Where, Why, and How. Identify a specific milestone you would like to reach and include the details needed to establish a timeframe, location, purpose, or benefit for the goal. *For example, a general goal might be "lose weight" but a specific goal would be "Workout three days a week".*

Measurable – It is essential that you establish specific criteria for measuring your success toward a particular goal. *For example, a general goal might be "lose weight" but a specific goal would be to "lose ten pounds this month".*

Attainable – Do not limit yourself or your dreams but keep in mind that the goals you set need to be practical and attainable. *For example, you might love the idea of losing 50 pounds in 50 days, but that may not be possible. Instead, set an attainable goal like "lose 50 pounds in 6 months".* You can always reach your goal before the proposed timeline.

Realistic – It is important to set lofty goals for yourself so that you are challenged to reach them, but you also need to set mid-range goals along the way. *For example, you might set a general goal to "lose 50 pounds" but you should set smaller realistic goals along the way like "lose two pounds per week".*

Timely – No matter what goals you set, you need to set a timeframe to create a sense of urgency and to motivate yourself to actually work toward that goal. *For example, you may want to reach your total goal of losing 50 pounds in 6 months and you can set smaller goals along the way like "lose 5 pounds the first week" or "lose 10 pounds per month".*

WHAT DOES SUCCESS LOOK LIKE TO YOU?

As you work on developing some SMART goals you need to think about what success looks like to you. For some people, success is all about shedding fat and reaching a specific goal weight. For others, it may be more important to increase physical fitness and to improve nutrition. You can customize your own journey in whatever way you like, just be sure to set tangible goals for yourself.

ACTION STEP #5

Set some SMART goals for yourself and stay motivated! By now you should have all of the tools you need to improve your nutrition, increase your activity level, and set some realistic goals. Now is the perfect time to take some measurements and "before" pictures of yourself. Believe me, you'll want them later when you fulfill your first goal and you want to see how far you've come! Follow the tips provided in this chapter to set a few SMART goals for yourself and then take the necessary steps to meet them.

CHAPTER 7. PALEO MEAL PLANS AND RECIPES FOR SUCCESS

By now you should have a deeper understanding of the importance of quality nutrition and the role it will play in helping you to reach your goal. Eating healthy is not as difficult or expensive as many people imagine it to be – all you have to do is stock up on some healthy foods when they go on sale and then make smart choices!

As simple as the Paleo diet is, it may still take you some time to get used to it. In this chapter you will find some useful resources to help you get started with the diet. Here you will find a simple Paleo meal plan for seven days which includes breakfast options, snacks, entrees, and even a few desserts. After following this meal plan for a week you should have a better understanding of the Paleo diet and you'll be able to customize the plan for continued use in the future.

SIMPLE PALEO MEAL PLAN

Following the Paleo diet does not necessarily mean that you have to cook every day. If you like cooking, of course, it is definitely an option. But many people simply do not have the time to prepare a fresh meal every day. The seven-day meal plan provided in this section is a blend of homemade recipes, simple snacks, and creative ways to use leftovers. With this meal plan in hand you should have no trouble making it through your first week on the Paleo diet. Once you make it through the first seven days the rest will be much easier.

			Sample 7-Day Paleo Meal Plan		
Day	**Breakfast**	**Snack**	**Lunch**	**Snack**	**Dinner**
1	Tomato, Onion and Basil Omelet	Fresh Fruit	Creamy Carrot Ginger Soup	Avocado Chocolate Mousse	Balsamic Grilled Chicken Breast with Steamed Veggies
2	Scrambled Eggs with Bacon	Dried Fruit and Nut Bar	Green Salad with Leftover Chicken	Fresh Sliced Veggies	Baked Halibut with Mango Salsa
3	Triple Berry Mint Smoothie	Salted Zucchini Chips	Chilled Avocado Soup	Fresh Fruit	Garlic Herb Turkey Burgers
4	Cinnamon Banana Pancakes	Fresh Fruit	Reheated Turkey Burger over Green Salad	Baked Sweet Potato Fries	Grilled Fish with Steamed Veggies
5	Scrambled Eggs with Sausage	Fresh Sliced Veggies	Roasted Tomato Basil Soup	Raspberry Beet Ginger Smoothie	Rosemary Roasted Chicken with Veggies
6	Spinach Kiwi Lime Smoothie	Vanilla Chia Seed Pudding	Chopped Chicken Pecan Salad	Fresh Fruit	Herb-Roasted Pork Tenderloin

7	Eggs Baked in Red Peppers	Fresh Fruit	Leftover Pork with Green Salad	Blueberry Coconut Smoothie	Slow-Cooker Pot Roast

SAMPLE PALEO DIET RECIPES

Recipes Included in this Book:

- Tomato, Onion and Basil Omelet
- Cinnamon Banana Pancakes
- Eggs Baked in Red Peppers
- Coconut Flour Blueberry Muffins
- Mushroom and Onion Frittata
- Pumpkin Cinnamon Waffles
- Diced Ham and Veggie Omelet
- Lemon Coconut Muffins
- Triple Berry Mint Smoothie
- Avocado Lime Walnut Smoothie
- Spinach Kiwi Lime Smoothie
- Raspberry Beet Ginger Smoothie
- Blueberry Coconut Smoothie
- Baked Sweet Potato Fries
- Dried Fruit and Nut Bars
- Salted Zucchini Chips
- Avocado Chocolate Mousse
- Strawberry Applesauce
- Vanilla Chia Seed Pudding
- Creamy Carrot Ginger Soup
- Spinach Salad with Balsamic Dressing
- Chopped Chicken Pecan Salad
- Roasted Tomato Basil Soup

- Lobster Avocado Salad
- Cauliflower Sweet Potato Soup
- Balsamic Grilled Chicken Breasts
- Slow-Cooker Pot Roast
- Baked Halibut with Mango Salsa
- Rosemary Roasted Chicken and Veggies
- Herb-Roasted Pork Tenderloin
- Garlic Herb Turkey Burgers
- Fried Salmon Sweet Potato Cakes
- Spaghetti Squash with Sautéed Veggies

Breakfast Recipes

Tomato, Onion and Basil Omelet

Servings: 1

Ingredients:

- 2 teaspoons olive oil
- 1 small tomato, diced
- 2 to 3 tablespoons diced white onion
- 1 clove minced garlic
- 2 large eggs, whisked well
- 1 tablespoon fresh chopped chives
- Salt and pepper to taste
- 2 tablespoons fresh chopped basil

Instructions:

1. Heat 1 teaspoon olive oil in a small skillet over medium heat.

2. Add the tomato, onion, and garlic then cook for 2 to 3 minutes until just tender.
3. Spoon the vegetables off into a bowl then reheat the skillet with the remaining oil.
4. Beat the eggs together with the chives, salt and pepper then pour them into the skillet.
5. Cook the eggs for one to two minutes without disturbing.
6. Use a spatula to lift the edges of the egg, allowing any uncooked egg to spread underneath.
7. Once the egg is almost set, spoon the vegetables over half of the omelet then sprinkle with basil.
8. Fold the omelet over the filling and cook for 30 to 60 seconds more until the egg is set.
9. Slide the omelet onto a plate and serve hot.

Cinnamon Banana Pancakes

Servings: 2 to 3

Ingredients:

- 4 large very ripe bananas, peeled and chopped
- 6 large eggs, whisked lightly
- ½ teaspoon baking powder
- 1 teaspoon vanilla extract
- ½ to 1 teaspoon ground cinnamon

Instructions:

1. Mash the bananas in a medium mixing bowl with a fork.

2. Stir in the eggs, baking powder, vanilla extract, and cinnamon.
3. Heat a large nonstick skillet over medium heat and grease it with olive oil cooking spray.
4. Spoon the batter into the skillet, using about 2 to 3 tablespoons per pancake.
5. Cook the pancakes until the underside is just browned.
6. Carefully flip the pancakes and cook for another minute or two until browned underneath.
7. Remove the pancakes to a plate to keep warm and repeat with the remaining batter.
8. Serve the pancakes warm drizzled with raw honey or maple syrup.

Eggs Baked in Red Peppers

Servings: 4

Ingredients:

- 4 red bell peppers
- 1 tablespoon coconut oil
- 1 medium yellow onion, diced
- 1 ½ cups sliced mushrooms
- 1 medium stem tomato, diced
- 1 clove minced garlic
- Salt and pepper to taste
- 8 large eggs, beaten well
- Fresh chopped parsley

Instructions:

1. Preheat the oven to 375°F.
2. Cut the peppers in half lengthwise and remove the core and seeds.
3. Heat the coconut oil in a large skillet over medium heat.
4. Add the onion and cook for 3 to 4 minutes until soft.
5. Stir in the mushrooms, tomatoes, and garlic then cook for 2 to 3 minutes until tender.
6. Season the vegetables with salt and pepper to taste.
7. Spoon the vegetable mixture into the red peppers then place them upright in a large baking dish.
8. Beat the eggs with some salt and pepper then pour the mixture into the peppers.
9. Bake the peppers for 35 to 40 minutes until the egg is set then serve hot garnished with fresh parsley.

Coconut Flour Blueberry Muffins

Servings: 12

Ingredients:

- 1 cup sifted coconut flour
- ¾ teaspoon baking soda
- ½ teaspoon salt
- 6 large eggs, whisked well
- ½ cup coconut oil, melted
- ½ cup pure maple syrup
- ½ tablespoon vanilla extract
- 1 cup fresh blueberries

Instructions:

1. Preheat the oven to 350°F and line a muffin pan with paper liners.
2. Combine the coconut flour, baking soda and salt in a medium mixing bowl.
3. In a separate bowl, whisk together the eggs, coconut oil, maple syrup and vanilla.
4. Whisk the wet ingredients into the dry until smooth and well combined then fold in the blueberries.
5. Spoon the batter into the prepared pan, filling the cups about ½ full.
6. Bake for 20 to 25 minutes until a knife inserted in the center of a muffin comes out clean.
7. Cool the muffins for 5 minutes in the pan then turn them out onto a wire rack to cool completely.

Mushroom and Onion Frittata

Servings: 4

Ingredients:

- 2 tablespoons coconut oil
- 1 small yellow onion, chopped
- 8 to 10 ounces sliced mushrooms
- Salt and pepper to taste
- 3 to 4 cups fresh chopped spinach
- 8 large eggs, beaten well

Instructions:

1. Preheat the broiler in your oven to high heat.

2. Melt the coconut oil in a large oven-safe skillet over medium-high heat.
3. Add the onions and cook for 4 to 6 minutes until tender.
4. Stir in the mushrooms then season with salt and pepper to taste.
5. Cook the mushrooms for 6 to 7 minutes until most of the liquid has cooked off.
6. Stir in the spinach and cook until just wilted, about 1 to 2 minutes.
7. Spread the vegetable mixture evenly in the bottom of the skillet.
8. Pour in the beaten eggs and spread evenly.
9. Cook the frittata on the stovetop on medium-high heat for 6 to 7 minutes until the bottom is just set.
10. Transfer the frittata to the oven and broil for 6 to 7 minutes until the egg is set and the top is browned.
11. Remove the frittata from the oven and let cool for a few minutes before slicing to serve.

Pumpkin Cinnamon Waffles

Servings: 4 to 6

Ingredients:

- ½ cup pureed pumpkin
- ¼ cup canned coconut milk
- 2 large eggs, whisked well
- 2 tablespoons raw honey
- 1 teaspoon vanilla extract

- ¾ cups blanched almond flour
- ½ cup shredded unsweetened coconut
- 1 teaspoon ground cinnamon
- Pinch ground nutmeg
- Pinch salt

Instructions:

1. Preheat your waffle iron and grease with olive oil cooking spray.
2. Combine the pumpkin, coconut milk, eggs, honey and vanilla extract in a mixing bowl.
3. In a separate bowl whisk together the almond flour, coconut, cinnamon, nutmeg and salt.
4. Stir the dry ingredients into the wet ingredients until smooth and well combined – add more coconut milk if needed to blend.
5. Spoon the mixture into your waffle iron, using about ¼ to ½ cup per waffle.
6. Close the waffle iron and cook until the waffle is crisp and browned.
7. Transfer the waffle to a plate to keep warm and repeat with the remaining batter.
8. Serve the waffles warm drizzled with honey or maple syrup.

Diced Ham and Veggie Omelet

Servings: 1

Ingredients:

- 2 teaspoons olive oil
- ½ small yellow onion, diced
- ¼ cup diced mushrooms
- ¼ cup diced zucchini
- 1 clove minced garlic
- 2 large eggs, whisked well
- 1 tablespoon sliced green onion
- Salt and pepper to taste
- 1 tablespoons fresh chopped parsley

Instructions:

1. Heat 1 teaspoon olive oil in a small skillet over medium heat.
2. Add the onion, mushrooms, zucchini, and garlic then cook for 2 to 3 minutes until just tender.
3. Spoon the vegetables off into a bowl then reheat the skillet with the remaining oil.
4. Beat the eggs together with the green onion, salt and pepper then pour them into the skillet.
5. Cook the eggs for one to two minutes without disturbing.
6. Use a spatula to lift the edges of the egg, allowing any uncooked egg to spread underneath.
7. Once the egg is almost set, spoon the vegetables over half of the omelet then sprinkle with parsley.

8. Fold the omelet over the filling and cook for 30 to 60 seconds more until the egg is set.
9. Slide the omelet onto a plate and serve hot.

Lemon Coconut Muffins

Servings: 12

Ingredients:

- 1 cup sifted coconut flour
- 1 teaspoon baking soda
- ½ teaspoon salt
- 6 large eggs, whisked well
- ½ cup coconut oil, melted
- ½ cup raw honey
- 1 tablespoon fresh lemon zest
- ½ cup shredded unsweetened coconut

Instructions:

1. Preheat the oven to 350°F and line a muffin pan with paper liners.
2. Combine the coconut flour, baking soda and salt in a medium mixing bowl.
3. In a separate bowl, whisk together the eggs, coconut oil, honey and lemon zest.
4. Whisk the wet ingredients into the dry until smooth and well combined then fold in the shredded coconut.
5. Spoon the batter into the prepared pan, filling the cups about ½ full.

6. Bake for 20 to 25 minutes until a knife inserted in the center of a muffin comes out clean.
7. Cool the muffins for 5 minutes in the pan then turn them out onto a wire rack to cool completely.

Triple Berry Mint Smoothie

Servings: 1

Ingredients:

- 1 cup frozen blueberries
- ½ cup frozen sliced strawberries
- ¼ cup frozen raspberries
- ½ small frozen banana, peeled and sliced
- 1 cup unsweetened almond milk
- ½ cup ice cubes
- ½ cup fresh chopped mint
- 1 teaspoon raw honey (optional)

Instructions:

1. Combine all of the ingredients in a high-speed blender.
2. Pulse the ingredients several times to chop them.
3. Blend on high speed for 30 to 60 seconds until smooth and well combined – add more liquid if needed to thin.

4. Pour the smoothie into a large glass and enjoy immediately.

Avocado Lime Walnut Smoothie

Servings: 1

Ingredients:

- ½ ripe avocado, pitted and chopped
- 1 small frozen banana, peeled and sliced
- 1 handful fresh spinach
- 1 cup canned coconut milk
- ½ cup ice cubes
- 1 ripe lime, juiced
- 1 teaspoon lime zest
- 2 tablespoons chopped walnuts

Instructions:

1. Combine all of the ingredients in a high-speed blender.
2. Pulse the ingredients several times to chop them.
3. Blend on high speed for 30 to 60 seconds until smooth and well combined – add more liquid if needed to thin.
4. Pour the smoothie into a large glass and enjoy immediately.

Spinach Kiwi Lime Smoothie

Servings: 1

Ingredients:

- 1 ½ cups fresh chopped spinach
- 1 small frozen banana, peeled and sliced
- 2 ripe kiwi, peeled and sliced
- 1 cup unsweetened almond milk
- ½ cup ice cubes
- 2 tablespoons fresh lime juice
- 1 teaspoon raw honey

Instructions:

1. Combine all of the ingredients in a high-speed blender.
2. Pulse the ingredients several times to chop them.
3. Blend on high speed for 30 to 60 seconds until smooth and well combined – add more liquid if needed to thin.
4. Pour the smoothie into a large glass and enjoy immediately.

Raspberry Beet Ginger Smoothie

Servings: 1

Ingredients:

- 2 cups frozen raspberries
- 1 small carrot, peeled and chopped

- 1 small beet, scrubbed and chopped
- 1 cup unsweetened apple juice
- 1 inch fresh chopped ginger
- 1 teaspoon raw honey

Instructions:

1. Combine all of the ingredients in a high-speed blender.
2. Pulse the ingredients several times to chop them.
3. Blend on high speed for 30 to 60 seconds until smooth and well combined – add more liquid if needed to thin.
4. Pour the smoothie into a large glass and enjoy immediately.

Blueberry Coconut Smoothie

Servings: 1

Ingredients:

- 1 ½ cups frozen blueberries
- 1 small frozen banana, peeled and sliced
- 1 handful fresh spinach
- 1 cup unsweetened coconut milk
- ½ cup ice cubes
- 2 tablespoons shredded unsweetened coconut
- Pinch ground cinnamon

Instructions:

1. Combine all of the ingredients in a high-speed blender.
2. Pulse the ingredients several times to chop them.
3. Blend on high speed for 30 to 60 seconds until smooth and well combined – add more liquid if needed to thin.
4. Pour the smoothie into a large glass and enjoy immediately.

Baked Sweet Potato Fries

Servings: 4

Ingredients:

- 4 large sweet potatoes
- 1 to 2 tablespoons olive oil
- 1 teaspoon chili powder
- ½ teaspoon smoked paprika
- Salt and pepper to taste

Instructions:

1. Preheat the oven to 450°F and line a baking sheet with parchment paper.
2. Peel the sweet potatoes and cut them into sticks or wedges, as desired.
3. Place the sweet potatoes in a large bowl and drizzle with olive oil.
4. Toss the sweet potatoes with the chili powder, paprika, salt and pepper.

5. Spread the sweet potatoes on the baking sheet in a single layer.
6. Bake for 18 to 22 minutes until tender and browned.
7. Let the fries cool for 5 to 10 minutes then serve warm.

Dried Fruit and Nut Bars

Servings: 8

Ingredients:

- 1 ½ cups raw almonds
- ½ cup walnut halves
- 2 cups pitted Medjool dates
- 1 cup dried pitted cherries
- 1 cup dried cranberries or raisins
- ¼ teaspoon ground cinnamon
- Pinch ground nutmeg

Instructions:

1. Preheat your oven to 400°F.
2. Spread the almonds and walnuts on a rimmed baking sheet and bake for 8 to 10 minutes until toasted.
3. Let the nuts cool then add them to a food processor.
4. Add the remaining ingredients and pulse them to chop.
5. Keep pulsing the mixture together until it forms a sticky mixture that comes together.
6. Line a baking sheet with parchment and turn the fruit and nut mixture out onto it.

7. Shape the mixture by hand into a rectangle then cover with parchment and chill for 2 hours.
8. Cut the mixture into eight even-sized bars.

Salted Zucchini Chips

Servings: 4

Ingredients:

- 2 large zucchini
- 2 teaspoons olive oil
- Salt to taste

Instructions:

1. Use a mandolin to slice the zucchini as thin as possible.
2. Spread the zucchini slices out on paper towel and sprinkle with salt.
3. Let the slices rest for 20 minutes then pat dry with clean paper towels.
4. Preheat the oven to 230°F.
5. Transfer the slices to a parchment-lined baking sheet and brush with oil.
6. Bake the zucchini slices for 2 ½ hours until crisp then sprinkle lightly with salt to serve.

Avocado Chocolate Mousse

Servings: 4

Ingredients:

- 2 large ripe avocadoes, pitted and chopped
- ¼ to ½ cup unsweetened cocoa powder
- 2 tablespoons raw honey
- 1 to 2 tablespoons almond butter
- Pinch salt

Instructions:

1. Place the chopped avocado in a food processor.
2. Add the cocoa powder, honey, almond butter, and salt.
3. Blend the ingredients until smooth and well combined.
4. Spoon the mousse into dessert cups and chill for at least 1 hour before serving.

Strawberry Applesauce

Servings: 4 to 6

Ingredients:

- 5 lbs. ripe apples, peeled, cored, and diced
- 15 large strawberries, stems removed
- 4 to 6 tablespoons raw honey
- ¼ cup fresh lemon juice
- 1 teaspoon vanilla extract

- ½ teaspoon ground cinnamon

Instructions:

1. Chop the apples and strawberries into small pieces then combine them in a large saucepan.
2. Stir in the honey, lemon juice, vanilla, and cinnamon.
3. Bring the mixture to a boil then reduce heat and simmer for 35 to 45 minutes until the apples are very tender.
4. Transfer the mixture to a food processor and blend smooth.
5. Chill the applesauce, if desired, before serving.

Vanilla Chia Seed Pudding

Servings: 4

Ingredients:

- ¾ cups raw chia seeds
- 3 cups unsweetened almond milk
- 1 tablespoon vanilla extract
- 2 tablespoons raw honey
- ¼ teaspoon ground cinnamon
- Fresh fruit, as desired

Instructions:

1. Combine the chia seeds, almond milk, and vanilla extract in a medium bowl.
2. Whisk in the honey and ground cinnamon.
3. Cover the bowl and let it chill overnight.

4. Spoon the pudding into cups and serve with fresh chopped fruit.

Soups and Salads

Creamy Carrot Ginger Soup

Servings: 4 to 6

Ingredients:

- 1 tablespoon coconut oil
- 1 medium yellow onion, chopped
- 2 tablespoons fresh grated ginger
- 2 cloves minced garlic
- 10 large carrots, peeled and chopped
- 1 small zucchini, chopped
- 1 medium ripe apple, cored and chopped
- 1 teaspoon ground cinnamon
- 5 cups chicken stock
- 1 cup canned coconut milk
- Salt and pepper to taste

Instructions:

1. Heat the oil in a large saucepan over medium-high heat.
2. Add the onion, ginger and garlic then cook for 4 to 5 minutes until tender.
3. Stir in the remaining vegetables along with the apple and cinnamon.

4. Pour in the chicken stock then bring the mixture to a boil.
5. Reduce heat and simmer for 25 to 30 minutes until the vegetables are very tender.
6. Remove from heat then puree the soup using an immersion blender until smooth.
7. Return to heat and whisk in the coconut milk.
8. Season with salt and pepper to taste then serve hot.

Spinach Salad with Balsamic Dressing

Servings: 4

Ingredients:

- 6 cups fresh baby spinach, packed
- 1 ½ cups sliced mushrooms
- ¼ cup thinly sliced red onion
- ¼ cup olive oil
- 2 tablespoons balsamic vinegar
- 1 tablespoon Dijon mustard
- 1 teaspoon raw honey
- Pinch salt and pepper
- 2 to 3 tablespoons toasted sunflower seeds

Instructions:

1. Combine the spinach, mushrooms, and red onion in a large salad bowl.
2. Toss well then divide the salad among four salad bowls.

3. Whisk together the remaining ingredients in a small bowl.
4. Drizzle the dressing over the salads then garnish with toasted sunflower seeds to serve.

Chopped Chicken Pecan Salad

Servings: 8 to 10

Ingredients:

- 2 large boneless skinless chicken breasts, cooked
- 1 cup toasted pecans, chopped
- 2 stalks celery, diced small
- 1 small green apple, cored and diced
- ½ cup dried cranberries
- 2 tablespoons minced red onion
- 1 large egg, whisked well
- 1 teaspoon fresh lemon juice
- 1 teaspoon Dijon mustard
- 1 teaspoon raw honey (optional)
- ½ to 2/3 cups olive oil
- Salt and pepper to taste
- Chopped lettuce, to serve

Instructions:

1. Shred the chicken by hand into a large bowl.
2. Toss in the pecans, celery, apple, cranberries, and red onion.
3. Whisk together the egg, lemon juice, mustard, and honey in a medium mixing bowl.

4. While whisking, drizzle in the olive oil until the mixture thickens.
5. Season with salt and pepper to taste.
6. Toss the homemade mayonnaise with the salad mixture until it reaches the desired consistency.
7. Serve the chicken salad over chopped lettuce.

Roasted Tomato Basil Soup

Servings: 4 to 6

Ingredients:

- 6 medium ripe tomatoes, cored and quartered
- 1 large yellow onion, sliced thick
- 6 cloves fresh garlic, peeled and sliced
- 1 to 2 tablespoons olive oil
- Salt and pepper to taste
- 2 cups vegetable stock
- ½ cup fresh chopped basil
- ½ cup canned coconut milk

Instructions:

1. Preheat the oven to 350°F.
2. Spread the tomatoes, onions, and garlic on a rimmed baking sheet.
3. Drizzle with olive oil then season with salt and pepper to taste.
4. Roast the vegetables for 35 to 40 minutes until lightly charred, tossing once halfway through.

5. Transfer the vegetables to a large saucepan then stir in the vegetable stock and basil.
6. Bring the mixture to a boil then reduce heat and simmer for 5 minutes.
7. Remove from heat and puree the soup using an immersion blender.
8. Return to heat and whisk in the coconut milk.
9. Adjust seasonings to taste and serve hot.

Lobster Avocado Salad

Servings: 4 to 6

Ingredients:

- 5 (8-ounce) lobster tails, thawed if frozen
- ½ cup canned coconut milk
- 2 tablespoons fresh lemon juice
- 1 teaspoon Dijon mustard
- Salt and pepper to taste
- 1 large ripe avocado, pitted and diced
- 2 stalks celery, diced small
- ¼ cup diced red onion
- 2 to 3 tablespoons fresh chopped cilantro
- Salt and pepper to taste

Instructions:

1. Bring a large pot of salted water to a boil.
2. Add the lobster tails to the boiling water then cover with the lid.

3. Boil the lobster tails for 8 to 10 minutes until the shells are bright red.
4. Drain the lobster tails and rinse well with cool water to stop the cooking.
5. Remove the meat from the lobster tails and chop into bite-sized pieces.
6. In a large mixing bowl, whisk together the coconut milk, lemon juice, Dijon mustard, salt and pepper.
7. Toss in the chopped lobster along with the avocado, celery, red onion, and cilantro.
8. Season the salad with salt and pepper to taste then chill for at least 1 hour before serving.

Cauliflower Sweet Potato Soup

Servings: 4 to 6

Ingredients:

- 1 medium head cauliflower, chopped
- 2 large sweet potatoes, peeled and chopped
- 1 small yellow onion, chopped
- 6 cloves garlic, peeled and sliced
- 2 to 3 tablespoons olive oil
- Salt and pepper to taste
- 5 cups chicken stock
- ½ cup canned coconut milk

Instructions:

1. Preheat the oven to 400°F.

2. Toss together the cauliflower, sweet potato, onions, and garlic on a rimmed baking sheet.
3. Drizzle with olive oil then season with salt and pepper to taste.
4. Roast the vegetables for 35 to 40 minutes until tender, tossing once halfway through.
5. Spoon the roasted vegetables into a large saucepan.
6. Pour in the stock then bring the mixture to a boil.
7. Reduce heat and simmer for 5 minutes.
8. Remove from heat and puree the soup using an immersion blender.
9. Return to heat and whisk in the coconut oil then season with salt and pepper to taste. Serve hot.

MAIN ENTRÉE RECIPES

Balsamic Grilled Chicken Breasts

Servings: 6

Ingredients:

- 1/3 cup olive oil
- 1/3 cup balsamic vinegar
- 1 tablespoon minced garlic
- 1 tablespoon Dijon mustard
- Salt and pepper to taste
- 2 pounds boneless skinless chicken breast halves

Instructions:

1. Whisk together the olive oil, balsamic vinegar, garlic, Dijon mustard, salt and pepper in a small bowl.
2. Trim the fat from the chicken breast halves then place them in a shallow dish.
3. Pour the marinade over the chicken, turning to coat, then cover with plastic and chill for at least 1 hour.
4. Preheat the grill to high heat and brush the grates with olive oil.
5. Place the chicken breast halves on the grill and cook for 5 to 6 minutes on each side until the internal temperature reaches 165°F.
6. Transfer the chicken breasts to a cutting board and let rest 5 minutes before slicing to serve.

Slow-Cooker Pot Roast

Servings: 6

Ingredients:

- 2 tablespoons coconut oil
- 1 (4 to 4 ½ pound) boneless beef chuck roast
- Salt and pepper to taste
- 4 large carrots, peeled and sliced
- 2 medium turnips, peeled and sliced
- 2 medium parsnips, peeled and sliced
- 1 large onion, quartered
- 3 cloves fresh minced garlic
- 1 tablespoon fresh chopped thyme
- 2 small bay leaves
- 2 ½ cups beef broth or stock

- Up to ¼ cup tapioca flour

Instructions:

1. Heat the coconut oil in a large skillet over medium heat.
2. Trim the fat from the roast and season with salt and pepper to taste.
3. Place the roast in the preheated skillet and cook for 2 to 3 minutes on each side until seared.
4. Combine the carrots, turnips, parsnips and onion in the slow cooker.
5. Place the roast on top of the vegetables then sprinkle with garlic, thyme, salt and pepper.
6. Add the bay leaves and pour in the beef stock.
7. Cover the slow cooker and cook on low heat for 8 hours until the roast is very tender.
8. Remove the roast to a cutting board and cover with foil to keep warm.
9. Spoon the vegetables into a large bowl to keep warm.
10. Discard the bay leaf then puree the mixture left in the slow cooker using an immersion blender.
11. Pour the mixture into a medium saucepan and cook over medium heat.
12. Whisk in the tapioca flour a teaspoon at a time and simmer the mixture until thick.
13. Serve the pot roast hot with veggies, drizzled with the hot gravy.

Baked Halibut with Mango Salsa

Servings: 4

Ingredients:

- 4 (6-ounce) boneless halibut fillets
- 1 tablespoon olive oil
- Salt and pepper to taste
- 1 medium ripe mango, pitted and diced
- 1 small tomato, cored and diced
- ¼ cup fresh chopped cilantro
- 2 tablespoons minced red onion
- 1 teaspoon fresh lime juice
- Pinch cayenne pepper

Instructions:

1. Preheat the oven to 350°F.
2. Rinse the halibut fillets in cool water then pat dry with paper towels.
3. Brush the fillets with olive oil and season with salt and pepper then place them on a baking sheet lined with parchment.
4. Bake the fillets for 12 to 15 minutes until the flesh flakes easily with a fork.
5. While the fish is cooking, toss together the remaining ingredients to make the salsa.
6. Serve the fillets hot topped with mango salsa.

Rosemary Roasted Chicken and Veggies

Servings: 4 to 6

Ingredients:

- 8 to 10 chicken drumsticks
- Salt and pepper to taste
- 2 tablespoons coconut oil
- 2 medium sweet potatoes, cut into large chunks
- 1 large yellow onion, cut into large chunks
- 1 cup fresh chopped broccoli florets
- 1 cup fresh chopped cauliflower florets
- 2 large carrots, peeled and sliced
- ¼ cup chicken stock
- 2 tablespoons fresh chopped rosemary

Instructions:

1. Preheat the oven to 400°F.
2. Season the chicken with salt and pepper to taste.
3. Heat the coconut oil in a large skillet over medium-high heat.
4. Add the chicken to the skillet and cook for 2 to 3 minutes on each side until browned.
5. Combine the sweet potatoes, onions, broccoli, cauliflower and carrots in a large bowl.
6. Toss with olive oil until evenly coated then spread the vegetables in a rectangular glass baking dish.
7. Arrange the browned chicken drumsticks on top of the vegetables in a single layer skin-side down.
8. Drizzle with chicken stock and sprinkle with rosemary then roast for 30 minutes.

9. Turn the chicken drumsticks then roast for another 25 to 30 minutes until the juices run clear.
10. Let the chicken rest for 10 minutes then serve with the roasted vegetables.

Herb-Roasted Pork Tenderloin

Servings: 4 to 6

Ingredients:

- 1 (3 to 4 pound) boneless pork loin
- 2 tablespoons fresh chopped rosemary
- 2 tablespoons fresh chopped thyme
- 1 teaspoon fresh chopped oregano
- 4 cloves garlic, minced
- Salt and pepper to taste
- Olive oil, if needed

Instructions:

1. Preheat the oven to 350°F.
2. Combine the rosemary, thyme, oregano, garlic, salt and pepper in a food processor.
3. Blend the mixture into a smooth paste, adding a little olive oil if needed.
4. Rub the garlic herb mixture into the pork tenderloin on all sides then place it in the middle of a roasting pan, fat-side up.
5. Roast for 60 minutes then check the internal temperature.

6. Cook the tenderloin for another 10 to 20 minutes until the internal temperature reaches 160°F.
7. Remove the pork to a cutting board and tent loosely with foil.
8. Let the pork rest for 10 minutes before slicing to serve.

Garlic Herb Turkey Burgers

Servings: 8

Ingredients:

- 1 tablespoon olive oil
- 1 small yellow onion, chopped
- 3 large cloves garlic, minced
- 2 pounds lean ground turkey breast
- ½ cup fresh chopped parsley
- ¼ cup fresh chopped cilantro
- 1 teaspoon fresh chopped rosemary
- 1 teaspoon fresh chopped sage
- Salt and pepper to taste

Instructions:

1. Heat the oil in a large skillet over medium heat.
2. Add the onion and garlic then cook for 4 to 6 minutes until the onion is very tender.
3. Remove from heat and let cool then spoon the mixture into a large mixing bowl.
4. Add the ground turkey, parsley, cilantro, rosemary and sage then season with salt and pepper to taste.

5. Mix the ingredients together well by hand then shape into 8 even-sized patties.
6. Preheat your grill to high heat and brush the grates with olive oil.
7. Place the turkey patties on the grill and cook for 5 to 6 minutes on each side until cooked through.
8. Serve the burgers over lettuce with your favorite burger toppings.

Fried Salmon Sweet Potato Cakes

Servings: 6 to 8

Ingredients:

- 3 medium sweet potatoes, peeled
- 3 (6-ounce) cans Alaskan salmon in water, drained
- 4 green onions, sliced thin
- 2 tablespoons fresh chopped dill
- 1 ½ tablespoons Dijon mustard
- 1 tablespoon fresh lemon juice
- Salt and pepper to taste
- ¼ cup coconut oil

Instructions:

1. Cut the sweet potatoes into quarters and place them in a medium saucepan.
2. Add enough water to cover the sweet potatoes by at least one inch.

3. Bring the water to boil over medium-high heat then reduce heat and simmer, covered, for 15 to 20 minutes until tender.
4. Drain the sweet potatoes and place them in a large bowl.
5. Mash the sweet potatoes with a potato masher or a fork.
6. Flake the salmon into the bowl with the mashed sweet potatoes.
7. Stir in the green onions and dill along with the Dijon mustard, lemon juice, salt and pepper.
8. Shape the mixture by hand into small patties about ½ inch thick.
9. Heat the coconut oil in a medium skillet over medium-high heat until very hot.
10. Add the patties and cook for 4 to 5 minutes on each side until the bottom is browned.
11. Drain the patties on paper towels and serve warm with lemon wedges.

Spaghetti Squash with Sautéed Veggies

Servings: 4

Ingredients:

- 1 large spaghetti squash
- 1 tablespoon coconut oil
- 1 medium yellow onion, chopped
- 1 small zucchini, diced
- 1 small red bell pepper, cored and diced

- 1 cup diced mushrooms
- 1 teaspoon minced garlic
- Salt and pepper to taste
- 1 to 2 tablespoons fresh lemon juice
- ¼ to ½ cup fresh chopped parsley

Instructions:

1. Preheat the oven to 375°F.
2. Cut the spaghetti squash in half lengthwise then scoop out and discard the seeds.
3. Place the squash halves cut-side down in a glass baking dish.
4. Pour in about ½ cup of water then bake the squash for 30 to 35 minutes until just tender.
5. Let the squash cool a little bit then shred the flesh into a bowl using a fork.
6. Heat the oil in large skillet over medium-high heat.
7. Add the onion and cook for 3 to 4 minutes until just tender.
8. Stir in the zucchini, red pepper, diced mushrooms, and garlic then season with salt and pepper to taste.
9. Sauté the vegetables for 5 to 6 minutes until tender then stir in the shredded spaghetti squash.
10. Stir in the lemon juice and fresh parsley then spoon into bowls to serve.

ACTION STEP #6

Commit to following the Paleo meal plan for 1 week. One week is just seven days and it is just enough time to get used to the basic principles of the Paleo diet. The meal plan included in this chapter is designed to be simple and easy to follow – you don't need any fancy ingredients and you won't have to spend hours cooking every day. Once you get the hang of the Paleo diet you can swap out some of the recipes in the meal plan for other recipes provided in this chapter or for recipes you find yourself. After you've made it through a few weeks on the Paleo diet you may be ready to branch out on your own or you can keep recycling the meal plan to keep yourself on track.

Chapter 8. Conclusion

After reading this book it is my hope that you come away knowing a few key things. For one thing, I hope you know that you are not alone. If you are overweight or obese and tired of the emotional and physical pain that entails, there are hundreds, even thousands (or millions) of people who feel the exact same way – and I was one of them! I know first-hand that changing your life is difficult, especially if you have a hundred or more pounds to lose. I also know first-hand, however, the power of self-motivation. If you believe that you can do something, you can!

I also hope that you come away from reading this book knowing that you are worth it. Even if the media (and sometimes your own friends and family) make you feel worthless or like less of a person because of your weight, I want you to know that it simply isn't true! The "old you" is still in there somewhere and you can bring him or her back with a little dedication and a lot of hard work.

If you are feeling a little bit overwhelmed at this point, I completely understand. I have given you a lot of information and I've covered several years of my life all in just a few pages. I want you to understand that it took time for me to get to where I am today, but I am so thankful that I made the choice to make a change. You have the power to change your habits and to transform your life and body. I believe in you and I hope you believe in yourself as well!

As you embark on your journey toward health and fitness you should expect to experience challenges along the way. There will be days where you are so sore that you can barely drag yourself out of bed. There will be days when all you want to do is chow down on a burger and fries. There will even be days where you wonder if all of the hard work is worth it. I want you to know that it is!

On those days where everything seems too hard or your goals seem too far away, I want you to picture yourself at the end of your journey. What do you look like? What kind of goals have you accomplished? In what ways has your life changed? If looking forward to the future isn't enough to motivate you to keep going, try looking back. Think about where you were when you first started your journey and remember all of the goals you have met to this point.

Even if you are only a few weeks in and you haven't lost a substantial amount of weight, you have probably gained some confidence in yourself. You have learned how to make healthier food choices and you have started to increase your activity level. Every victory counts, no matter how small.

As I think back on my own journey I am filled with excitement for you – and hope. I know that you have it in you to make the necessary changes to transform your life. I am living proof that obesity does not have to be a permanent condition. You can take back control of your life and transform your mind, body, and spirit. Renew your commitment to your journey and to yourself and go forth with confidence and pride!

Appendix: Action Step Summary and Helpful Forms

Action Step #1

Find what motivates you! List out your motivating factors, have you suffered emotional pain or physical pain like I have? Do you have children or want children some day and want to set a good example and be healthy enough to run around with them.

Have you had an unwelcome health event that may have been an eye opener to you?

Let me share with you a quote from one of my favorite Authors and Pod-casters **Dan Miller**.

"Perhaps the unwelcome event you've encountered is just an opportunity to help you know how to stand up stronger."

List as many motivating factors as you can for when times get tough, start with 3 before you move on with this book and continue to add to this list for when it feels like it is getting tough

1. _____

2. _____

3. _____

Action Step #2

Create your own dream board! Collect pictures, quotes, brochures, advertisements, anything that represents the end goal of your journey. Where do you see yourself at the end of your journey and what kind of things do you hope to do or achieve once you've reached it? Put all of the pictures together on a bulletin board and place it somewhere that you will see it every day. As you progress and start to accomplish small goals along the way you can add to the dream board.

Action Step #3

Take stock of your current eating habits. Now that you understand what clean eating is you should have a better idea of how your current eating habits might be negatively affecting your health. Keep track of all of the foods you eat over the course of one 24-hour period and then take a look at it to see just how many unhealthy foods you are eating on a regular basis. You may also want to clean out your kitchen and pantry, removing unhealthy foods and foods that trigger unhealthy habits.

Action Step #4

Stock your kitchen with healthy, Paleo-friendly foods! Now that you understand the basics of the Paleo diet and have received detailed food lists for what you should and should not be eating, you have the resources you need to restock your kitchen and pantry with Paleo-friendly foods.

Refer to the food lists above and head to the grocery store to stock up – be sure to eat something before you go because grocery shopping on an empty stomach often leads to impulse buys. Once you've stocked your Paleo kitchen you can take advantage of the recipes and meal plans provided at the end of this book!

Action Step #5

Commit to exercising three times per week. It is up to you how you want to structure your exercise plan but a good place to start is with three workouts per week, at least two of those workouts including strength training exercises. If you are new to exercise you may want to start small with three 30-minute walks per week until your cardiovascular fitness improves a little bit. Once you are able to handle longer periods of exercise you can start to work in more rigorous cardio sessions as well as strength training sessions.

Action Step #6

Set some SMART goals for yourself and stay motivated! By now you should have all of the tools you need to improve your nutrition, increase your activity level, and set some realistic goals. Now is the perfect time to take some measurements and "before" pictures of yourself. Believe me, you'll want them later when you fulfill your first goal and you want to see how far you've come! Follow the tips provided in this chapter to set a few SMART goals for yourself and then take the necessary steps to meet them.

Action Step #7

Commit to following the Paleo meal plan for 1 week. One week is just seven days and it is just enough time to get used to the basic principles of the Paleo diet. The meal plan included in this chapter is designed to be simple and easy to follow – you don't need any fancy ingredients and you won't have to spend hours cooking every day. Once you get the hang of the Paleo diet you can swap out some of the recipes in the meal plan for other recipes provided in this chapter or for recipes you find yourself. After you've made it through a few weeks on the Paleo diet you may be ready to branch out on your own or you can keep recycling the meal plan to keep yourself on track.

Step #3: Daily Food Intake Log
Date: _____

Breakfast_____

_____

Calories: _____

Lunch_____

_____

Calories: _____

Dinner_____

_____

Calories: _____

Snacks_____

_____

_____

Calories: _____

Total Daily Calorie Log			
Breakfast	**Lunch**	**Dinner**	**Snacks**
		Total:	

STEP #4: PALEO SHOPPING LIST

Produce:

Fruits

Apples
Avocado
Bananas
Blackberries
Blueberries
Cantaloupe
Cherries
Cranberries
Grapes
Grapefruit
Honeydew
Kiwi
Lemons
Limes
Mangos
Oranges
Peaches
Pears
Pineapple
Raspberries
Strawberries

Refrigerated:

Meat and Seafood

Eggs
Bacon
Beef
Chicken
Turkey
Fresh fish
Shrimp
Scallops

Frozen Foods:

Frozen vegetables
Frozen fish
Frozen meat
Frozen fruits

Vegetables

Acorn squash
Asparagus
Arugula
Beets
Bell peppers
Broccoli
Cabbage
Carrots
Cauliflower
Celery
Cucumber
Eggplant
Fresh herbs
Garlic
Ginger
Green beans
Kale
Lettuce
Mushrooms
Onions
Spinach
Sweet Potato
Tomatoes
Zucchini

Dried Goods:

Nuts and Seeds

Almonds
Almond butter
Cashews
Cashew butter
Chia seeds
Dates
Dried fruit
Pecans
Sesame seeds
Sunflower seeds
Tahini
Walnuts

Oils and Vinegar

Avocado oil
Apple cider vinegar
Balsamic vinegar
Coconut oil
Olive oil
Walnut oil

Baking Items

Almond flour
Baking soda
Cocoa powder (unsweetened)
Coconut flour
Coconut milk
Dried herbs and spices
Honey, raw
Maple syrup
Shredded coconut
Tapioca starch
Vanilla extract

Other

Beef broth
Chicken broth
Vegetable broth
Herbal tea
Fruit juice
Coffee
Olives

Canned tomatoes
Canned tuna
Coconut aminos
Mustard
Canned vegetables
Canned fruits

STEP #5: WORKOUT LOG

	Date	Date	Date
Week Start Weight:			
Week End Weight:			

Exercise Name	Sets	Reps	Wt.	Sets	Reps	Wt.	Sets	Reps	Wt.

Cardio Exercises	Time	Distance

Notes: _____
_____
_____
_____
_____

STEP #6: SMART GOAL SHEET

Specific-

Measurable-

Attainable-

Realistic-

TimeFrame-

Complete Goal:
By:

Complete Goal:
By:

Complete Goal:
By:

REFERENCES

"7 Reasons to Add Strength Training to Your Workout Routine." Everyday Health. <http://www.everydayhealth.com/fitness/add-strength-training-to-your-workout.aspx>

"17 Benefits of Eating Paleo." Paleo Grubs. <http://paleogrubs.com/paleo-benefits>

"About Adult BMI." Centers for Disease Control and Prevention. <http://www.cdc.gov/healthyweight/assessing/bmi/adult_bmi/index.html>

"Best Beginner Weight-Training Guide with Easy-to-Follow Workout." Bodybuilding.com. <http://www.bodybuilding.com/fun/beginner_weight_training.htm>

Clark, Bruce. "The American Diet: A Sweet Way to Die." Food Safety News. <http://www.foodsafetynews.com/2010/02/the-american-diet-a-sweet-way-to-die/#.VwaUDfkrIuU>

"Creating SMART Goals." Top Achievement. <http://topachievement.com/smart.html>

"Facts and Statistics." President's Council on Fitness, Sports and Nutrition. <http://www.fitness.gov/resource-center/facts-and-statistics/>

"Personal Goal Setting." Mind Tools. <https://www.mindtools.com/page6.html>

"Strength Training 101: Where Do I Start?" Nerd Fitness. <https://www.nerdfitness.com/blog/2014/01/14/strength-training-101-where-do-i-start/>

"StrongLifts 5x5." Stronglifts. <http://stronglifts.com/5x5/>

"The 5 Most Important Lifts to Master." Daily Burn. <http://dailyburn.com/life/fitness/most-important-strength-exercises/>

"The Hunter-Gatherer Diet: A Brief Paleo History." Paleo Planning. <http://paleoplanning.com/brief-paleo-diet-history/>

"The Sad Consequences of the Standard American Diet." Atkins.com. <https://www.atkins.com/how-it-works/library/articles/the-sad-consequences-of-the-standard-american-diet>

"The Typical American Diet is Our Biggest Enemy." Pritikin Longevity Center and Spa. <https://www.pritikin.com/your-health/healthy-living/eating-right/1789-american-diet-our-biggest-risk-factor-for-disease-disability-and-death.html>

Welland, Diane. "Seven Principles of Clean Eating." Cooking Light. <http://www.cookinglight.com/eating-smart/smart-choices/clean-eating>

"What Are the Health Risks of Overweight and Obesity?" National Heart, Lung, and Blood Institute. <https://www.nhlbi.nih.gov/health/health-topics/topics/obe/risks>

MEET THE MODELS

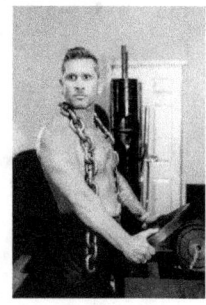

BRYAN E EIDEM

INBA Mr Reno sports model 2011,13,15

INBA/PNBA Coach of the year 2012

Fitness Trainer at BeeFitUSA.com

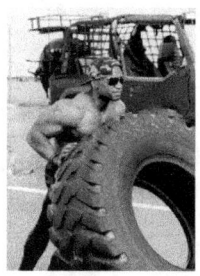

ROBERT DANIELS

Holds Professional status in PNBA and NGA

Winner of PNBA Team USA 2014

Natural Olympia Champion 2014 & 2015
RobertDanielsLifestyles.com

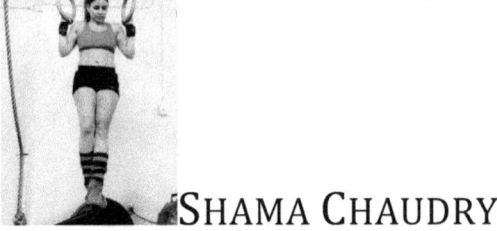

SHAMA CHAUDRY

INBA Fitness competitor & Fitness model

PHOTOGRAPHER

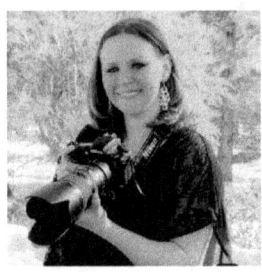

CASSANDRA R AARON

Traditional style wedding, portrait & event photographer in Reno, Nevada and the greater Lake Tahoe areas.

insideamomentphotography.com

ABOUT THE AUTHOR

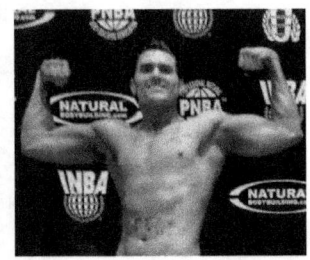

Derek A Cox has been a personal fitness trainer since 2005 when he received his first certification from the International Sports Science Association, Since then he has gone on to study Performance Nutrition, Fitness for Older Adults, Sports Performance, BioMarkers of Aging and Anti-Aging through Physical Training.

To further his education Derek has also taken many in depth classes that Include some studying under Dr. Dikito-Platz and her husband IFBB Pro hall of Fame Tom Platz on Natural Health, Applied Clinical Nutrition and Fitness training.

4th Place with over 80 athletes -Scottish Highlander Games

2nd Place Mr Nevada State -Natural Bodybuilding

3rd Place Team USA –Natural Bodybuilding

Team Trainer for 5 years Twin Cities Cougars Football Team

Learn More at DerekACox.com & FitBody2Go.com